ALSO BY JT LAWRENCE

THE
UNDERACHIEVING
OVARY

Will There Be Light at the End of the Birth Canal?

JT LAWRENCE

2016 Paperback edition

ISBN-13: 978-0-620-71673-4

Copyright © 2016 JT LAWRENCE

Published in South Africa by Pulp Books.

https://pulpbooks.wordpress.com

Book design by JT Lawrence

DEDICATION

This book is dedicated to my tribe
of fellow infertility warriors.

Also, to James, Robin, and Alexandra.
The love I have for you is infinite.

I

HEART-SHAPED HEARTBREAK

Today I was told that I have a heart-shaped uterus.

It sounds quirky, cute, but makes carrying a baby complicated. The sonar print-out is so pretty: a golden heart glowing from the static darkness. I lay there looking at the blizzard of a screen feeling a mixture of fascination and fear.

'Don't worry!' said the BFG (looking worried).

The BFG is my new gynae. I call him that after Roald Dahl's Big Friendly Giant. He is Dutch, taller than a doorframe, and extremely gentle. I can imagine him eating snozzcumbers behind his desk and blowing nice dreams into his patients' windows at night. What would they be about? Would they be gynaecologically themed? Maybe stories of perfect, cyst-free ovaries, like springy pink ping-pong balls, or fallopian tubes as open as the Chunnel. Perhaps in my case: a yawny old regular-shaped uterus. It would look boring on the outside, but would be totally pimped up on the inside - by the softest, most welcoming sticky red padding. Think diamond studs and dim lights. Bow-chicka-wow-wow.

'Don't worry!' he kept saying, making me worried. His Dutch accent reminded me of that Austin Powers character, Goldmember. I had to stop myself from asking, in what would be a terrible accent, if he would like a smoke and a pancake. No? Flapjack and a cigarette? Cigar and a waffle? Of course, Goldmember would have had problems having kids too, seeing as he lost his junk in an unfortunate smelting incident.

A heart-shaped uterus: surely it wasn't too much of a big deal? People come in all shapes and sizes, why would uteri be any different? Surely a bespoke uterus would be totally hip?

He finished the scan in silence and then, once I was dressed and back at his desk, he looked at me over steepled fingers. Blinked.

'Look,' he said.

FU-U-U-U-U-U-CK, I thought.

'It doesn't mean that you will *never* have children.'

My mind was blank at this point. Blind panic. I walked in here a healthy, fertile woman. Or what I thought was a healthy-ish, fertile-ish woman. If he had told me I had undescended testicles and an inside-out dick I couldn't have been more shocked.

I laughed. Of course I laughed. It was Laugh Or Die right there – keeling over on his uninspired carpet-tiled floor. I barked a short, humourless 'Gah!' and flicked my hair out of my hot face, as if to say: 'Of course it doesn't mean that I will never have children! I never thought that for a second!'

Because this isn't really happening, is it?

Wait. I had been fertile moments ago. What happened? I needed a rewind button, an Apple-Z.

'What does it mean?' I asked in my most grown-up voice, even though I felt like a bewildered little girl.

The BFG drew a messy heart on his prescription pad. An unlucky love letter. Underneath he scrawled 'BICORNIATE UTERUS'. He circled the twin tops of the heart.

'Bicorniate: two horns,' he explained.

My pretty heart-shaped organ just went from romantic baby chamber to devil-womb. It has more in common with bearded goats and demons than a symbol of affection.

'But what does it mean?' I asked again.

'You may find it ... difficult to fall pregnant. Basically, this part,' he said, dotting the cleft in the middle of the heart, 'gets in the way.'

I was too shocked to cry. Trust me to have an infernal uterus.

'But,' he smiled – the generous smile of a giant – 'you can still conceive. It's not impossible.'

I wish he hadn't used the word impossible. It's starting to sound harder and harder.

I left his office at the hospital and drove home on automatic pilot. Despite knowing exactly where I was going it was the most lost I've ever felt. Loneliest drive of my life. The doctor's words kept coming back to me.

I wondered how I would tell Mike. I would make him laugh first, offer him a pipe and a crêpe. Give him the unlucky love letter with the picture of the heart. Then tell him in the most reassuring way I could that he is married to someone who is harbouring a little (heart-shaped) pocket of Satan.

...

Later I dreamt that I gave birth to the devil's lovechild, Rosemary's-Baby style. The father, *El Diablo*, lost his temper and things exploded because he couldn't find his cigar. I wondered about his waffle. So much for the BFG's snozzcumbers and sweet dreams.

A Short Note on Dildo Cams

Dildo Cams, for those not in the know, are the sonar wands gynaes use to scan your babymaker. The men in white coats call them transvaginal ultrasounds. They roll a condom over it, squirt some lube out of what looks like a fish-'n-chips-shop squeezy vinegar bottle, and put it up your vajayjay (the wand, not the vinegar bottle). The first time this happens, if you are not *au fait* with dildo cams, it can be quite disconcerting. They should really come with a warning, perhaps in the form of a fun video.

2

SLIPPY-SLIDE OF DEATH

I've been Googling the hell out of 'bicorniate uterus'. The results: not pretty. It becomes clear that even if I do manage to beat the odds and conceive, most of my pregnancies will result in miscarriage. The cleft just isn't good at holding on to embryos – it's not made of the right tissue – so they'll implant and die, implant and die – if they implant at all. I think of the months we've been trying to fall pregnant and wonder how many times our cells have fused together to create a perfect little embryo, only to have it land on my slippy-slide of death.

If it does by some miracle land on happy endometrial tissue, implant and survive, it will probably end in a dangerously premature birth, as the cleft gets in the way of the baby growing and doesn't budge. What's up with you, Cleft? Why do you have to be a hater? Stubborn bastard two-faced heart-shape, I think. Acting all love-and-peace-forever but really being nothing but an inconsiderate asshole.

So I've been pre-programmed to miscarry. It would be easier, in a way, to accept a miscarriage if I knew there was something wrong with the foetus, as there often is. But mine will probably be perfectly healthy and I'll lose them anyway.

I cried tonight. I cried and cried, as if I had already lost my babies.

In a way, I suppose I have.

3

ALL OF A SUDDEN MY SHOULDER IS ON FIRE

There's something else. I wasn't going to get into it but it's getting worse every month. I hate telling people about it because they look at me as if I've just spoken in tongues and then licked their face. They take a step back, put a limp hand up, as if to say 'Oh, I just remembered, there is somewhere I'm supposed to be.' They get that faraway look in their eyes, as if they are thinking of meadows and waterfalls and just-brushed unicorns. And those are the doctors' reactions. Friends and family are less polite, putting their fingers in their ears and singing 'My Milkshakes Bring All the Boys to the Yard'.

Anyway, here it is: Ever since I've been off the pill, I get shoulder pain when I get my period. Yes, shoulder pain. And only ever in my right shoulder. Yes, I know it doesn't make sense. It's menstruation for fuck's sake, not a volleyball/tennis/shotput tournament.

It's there and it's real and it hurts like a motherfucker. Despite the intensity of the pain, it seemed so nonsensical that I ignored it for months, thinking it must be a bizarre coincidence. But 28 days, tick-tock click-clock and Bam! All of a sudden my shoulder is on fire. I saw doctors about it: they didn't have a clue what it could be. Kept asking me the same questions over and over as if to catch me out, like the detectives do on Law & Order. I had the feeling they wanted to send me for a psych evaluation. Most just shrugged, gave me scripts for painkillers, and a referral to yet another doctor. Honestly, who can blame them? I told them it hurts to breathe when I have my period. I would also diagnose myself as crackers. But here I am with this deep, terrible ache that no amount of psychoanalysis will cure.

I was in denial for the first few months, took a couple of painkillers and called it coincidence. But soon the pain started overtaking the ibuprofen and, on a particularly bad day, I found myself too sore to work sitting at my desk so took my laptop to bed. I typed into the Google search bar: "shoulder pain" "menstruation".

I thought the search engine would secretly snigger and try to correct my search, saying 'Did you mean "shoulder pain" "marathon", or "stomach pain" "menstruation"? Maybe "Shangri-La Meditation"?

But it didn't. Instead, up popped pages of listings of the symptoms of endometriosis. When I saw that ugly word again and again it was like I had stepped out of my body and floated above it. I knew what endometriosis meant: snarled up baby-making tubes. It is one of the very few words that scare the bejeezus out of me. Only one word

11

is more frightening and they happen to be (decidedly unsexy) bedfellows: Infertility.

It's one of those things you avoid reading about, talking about, thinking about, until it happens to you, or someone close to you: like cancer, birth defects, homelessness, or twerking. The very idea makes your subconscious squirm away and think of something less worrying: your bond repayments, your cholesterol, that new dent in your car. Your creepy ginger neighbour.

I don't know which was racing faster: my brain or my heart. Both stood to lose a great deal if my Dr Google pseudo-diagnosis was correct, and both knew as I read, that it was. Link after link described my symptoms exactly: a hot, intense pain focused in the shoulder that radiates down, into the upper arm and ribcage. A constant hum of pain that makes it sore to inhale, difficult to lie down, and almost impossible to sleep.

But why the shoulder, if the problem is with my babymaker? Extremely rare in a way I wouldn't exactly choose to be, it turns out I have a condition called diaphragmatic endometriosis. The rogue endometrial tissue attached to my diaphragm swells and bleeds every month, damaging the cells around it, causing lesions, inflammation and the sincere desire to saw my arm off.

It's referred pain, which makes it sound like it doesn't really exist. This sends me into a flurry of philosophical thought. If this pain doesn't 'exist' in my shoulder, then nothing I know is true. When it hurts, it's so damn tangible, it's just me and the pain. If it doesn't exist, then I don't exist. I hurt, therefore I am.

Oh, diaphragmatic endometriosis, I am just getting to know you, and I have the feeling we're going to have a long and severely unfulfilling relationship.

Diaphragmatic fucking endometriosis.

One in a brazillion people have it, and I seem to be one of them.

4

You're Not Supposed to be Reading This

Wait, wait, wait. I feel like we started off on the wrong foot (wrong ovary?)

Here I am gossiping about my designer uterus and describing the horrible, sticky story of my diaphragm without a thought for pleasantries or any kind of context. It's my personal diary. A journal I started to help me process the trauma of infertility. The reason I just launched into the nitty-gritties is because you're not supposed to be reading this.

5

BEHEAD THE BARBIES

When we were on our honeymoon I was so sublimely happy. Not because I was married (never been a huge fan of marriage in general – I don't see the point of signing a contract that encourages you to take your partner for granted), not because I was married to the very best person I could have imagined for myself (although it didn't hurt), and not because we were spending three weeks travelling through Italy, France and Spain (again, didn't hurt).

Okay, I was happy about all of the above. The buildings in Italy! The bread in France! The atmosphere in Spain! And, I'll admit, the holiday was legendary. But above all, the thing that was making my face shine was the knowledge in the back of my mind that in a month's time I would be off the pill and ready to start MAKING BABIES. Something I have wanted *my entire life*.

I was already broody in primary school. I think I might have been born broody, if that is possible. I used to cut out pictures of babies and pregnant women and file them. Once I kidnapped two baby dolls from my nursery school; named them Nadia and Devon, and took them everywhere I went in a cardboard suitcase. As you can imagine, it used to worry the fuck out of my mother.

'I love them so much,' I told my mom after stealing the dolls, 'I thought they were mine.'

When Nadia and Devon started falling apart at the seams I begged my parents to buy me a 'Newborn Baby'. Instead of a petite, pretty, rose-lipped doll, it was the size of a newborn, swollen, wrinkled, and a little ugly-monkey looking, just as real newborns are. Oh, how I *needed* one! I feel my jaws tensing now just thinking about it.

Behead the Barbies, cut off My Little Pony's mane and tail, unstuff the teddies, smash Castle Greyskull – I would have sold them all and more to get this precious bundle into my arms. My parents finally acquiesced and peeled off the fragrant pink banknotes. And how I loved that doll! I spent hours cradling it, smelling its sweet skin, staring into its sky-coloured marbles for eyes.

Looking back, I imagine the sleepless nights my mom must have had, worrying that her daughter would become a) a teenage mother, b) a kleptomaniac, or c) an abductor. Funny in the way that's not funny at all – that now, at thirty years old, it's become clear that having a baby isn't going to be the easiest thing for me to do. Sad-funny. On a bad day, not funny at all.

The origin of the word honeymoon is 'sweet month' – as in the first sweet month of marriage before you realise the magnitude of your foolishness. No one's feet smell in those first few weeks, no one fights, no one is too tired for foreplay. Things have changed, of course, now that everyone lives together before tying the knot. I guess honeymoons aren't as rosy (or deceptive) as they used to be. I had lived with Mike for seven years before we got married, so there were no surprises there, but like a 1940s bride, I pictured our future with (baby-shaped) stars in my eyes. And like that naïve bride who sets herself up for disappointment, the stars have fallen away, and shadows have taken their place.

6

THE YEAR TO GET PREGNANT

It's September 2009 and I'm remembering my birthday dinner earlier this year. Because this year is The Year To Get Pregnant, and 30 is A Good Age To Get Pregnant, my birthday was the perfect opportunity to toss my contraceptive pill. Freshly returned from Europe and full of optimism, I tossed the blister pack into the bin with a flourish. I felt grand. Mike looked a bit pale. He sat down and seemed to swallow a lot more than usual.

I understand his trepidation. Our friends with small children get so little sleep that it looks like they've been punched in the face. Apart from raccoon eyes, there is the distracted way they talk, as if they have ADHD: conversations are cut short, cups of coffee are left to get cold or are knocked over, usually both. They yawn about how wonderful it is to have kids, how much joy and meaning they bring into your life, but as you start to agree and tell them about your Plan To Get Pregnant they look panic-stricken, shake their frowns, and make the cutting-off-their-head gesture as ferociously as they can without their partner seeing.

'Life as you know it will be over,' said at least a dozen of them, while wiping chocolate/poo off the ceiling. 'But it's ... lovely,' say the rest.

'It's never a good time to have kids,' say the ones with vomit on their shoes who want you to hurry up and have them so that they can see how someone else's life sucks too.

So I'm thinking of my birthday dinner, and how much wine we all drank, and how much we laughed, and how generally balls-to-the-wall carefree we felt. (I notice now how there had been no parents at the table). I announced rather loudly that my pill had been artfully disposed of – not that I needed to, everyone at the table knew The Plan – and my friends were joking that I was so broody I'd be knocked up within the month. How we laughed.

7

MAKING BABIES

While we wait out the rest of our first year of trying to get knocked up (a whole year of trying? Seriously? Who is running this crack-snorting-orangutan circus of a universe?), I'm trying all the alternative options to traditional fertility treatment.

People on the interwebz swear that endo can be controlled with your diet and positive thinking. This includes giving up booze, caffeine, carbs, dairy, grains, sugar, preservatives, and pretty much all things edible. My desperation drives me to do unthinkable things. Only when I stumble upon a recipe for kale flakes do I realise that it has gone too far. It was an Oprah-like A-ha Moment. It was as if my spirit had been lifted out of my body and I was looking down at this (hungry) stranger staring blankly at the screen of her laptop. She may have been drooling a little. It was a moment of sheer clarity: I saw that I was lying in a gastronomical gutter of raw broccoli and spinach soup, a lick away from being lost forever. As a personal emergency intervention, I immediately went out and bought and ate an entire tub of chocolate and caramel ice cream.

But all is not lost on the airy-fairy hippie-junk front of alternative medicine. Just because I can't live without wine (and bread) (and chocolate) etc., it doesn't mean I can't try the other stuff. I am reading a book called 'Making Babies' by Jill Blakeway, who they call the Fertility Goddess of New York (I don't know exactly who 'they' are, but you get the idea). She is an acupuncturist and herbalist, and an 'empathic and intuitive practitioner of Chinese medicine'. I know, I know, she sounds dodgy to me, too. But I was won over by something she wrote somewhere on one of the thousands of websites I trawl, looking for some kind of answer, some kind of hope.

She wrote that for many fertility doctors the world over, IVF is an extremely effective tool. However, this leads to its overuse when often something a lot simpler, cheaper, and less invasive would do. For these doctors, she wrote, wielding this IVF hammer, every fertility problem begins looking like a nail.

She is not against IVF, she merely prefers a gentler approach – first getting the patient completely balanced in hormones and health – and then if there is still no success, going in with the big guns. It makes sense to me. I will try this balance thing. I've made an appointment with an acupuncturist who comes highly recommended. Even if it doesn't work, the needles will be good practice for IVF.

Too Selfish

Sometimes I wonder if I have done something to cause our fertility issues. Maybe I had an infection that I didn't know about and didn't treat. Maybe I spent too much time in the sauna one holiday. Maybe I smoked too much in my 20s. Maybe I partied too much in general. Maybe I'm not nice enough. Maybe I'm just too selfish.

I know that it's irrational. Fertility is not based on a merit (or de-merit) system. But the thoughts crawl along in front of me anyway, like fat toxic-green caterpillars. Crack babies are born all the time, I tell myself. There was one in the news last week. I would (I hope) make a better parent than someone who'd do that to their baby. It's not a competition, I say, but suddenly it feels like it is, and I've just been lapped by a crack addict.

Nothing Says Romance Like Charting Cervical Mucous

So Dr Google has taught me that you can tell when you are ovulating by inspecting your cervical mucous. At first I was, like, my cervical what-what? I don't think I have that.

They have handy acronyms for everything, thank heavens, and this in the TTC (Trying To Conceive) support forums is called CM for short. I like the acronyms. I don't know how many times I could type 'mucous' without throwing up a little in my mouth.

So your CM changes throughout your cycle, and

just as you ovulate it is supposed to get slightly sticky, so that you can stretch it between your thumb and your forefinger. I imagine poor desperate TTCers everywhere, hunched over the loo, trying to establish if their CM is 'the consistency of egg white' or not. I can't imagine it's very effective foreplay.

DIRTY TWIGS & WOOD PYGMIES

At the end of Blakeway's book, 'Making Babies' (she makes it sound so easy), she generously gives the readers her contact details and invites us to contact her with comments and questions. Now, I'm sure that the Fertility Goddess of New York will be very busy knocking people up all over the big apple, but I'm going to email her anyway.

Mine is an interesting case* (or so I've been told), so perhaps it will catch her eye.

* It sounds almost flattering, being told your case is rare or interesting; but, let me tell you, the last thing you want is doctors looking at you with a sparkle in their eye.

I wrote how I liked her philosophy and explained my situation as briefly as I could, and asked for her guidance. I figure she'll say (if she replies at all) that I should go the less invasive route. Try the programme in her book, find balance, be patient, and if that doesn't work, perhaps begin an AI/IUI (artificial/interuterine insemination) cycle. It makes me feel calm just writing that.

The acupuncture was weird, but okay. As a semi-rational person, I find it hard to believe that sticking some needles into your skin is going to do anything but, well, leave tiny little needle-holes.

'But Blakeway!' I kept telling myself. Trust those with experience. The acupuncturist was explaining each needle and its intended energy path as it went in. I wanted to tell her not to bother but I didn't want to be rude. Instead I pretended to listen and made a list in my head of the things I still had to get done that week. The needles left irritated patches, which pleased her. A reaction is good, she said. It means something is happening. I didn't want to burst her bubble by telling her that the patches were probably only because I have annoyingly sensitive skin.

She prescribed some Chinese medicine for me. I wouldn't usually be up for that kind of thing but I'm currently a little indoctrinated by Blakeway. Her success rate is astounding — something like 75% — way better than any fertility clinic in South Africa (or New York). She must be doing something right. I imagined the Chinese meds would look like a packet of dirty twigs, but when I was given them at the counter they were all in clinical plastic pill bottles: regular gel capsules, compressed powder pills, and a tall, clear dispenser of natural progesterone cream. Where were the mud and sticks? I wanted to ask. I was certain I'd have to drink a bitter tea made of forest leaf mould sourced in Papua New Guinea by wood pygmies but it turned out that all I had to do was pop a few pills on certain days of my cycle.

Despite having spent more than a thousand rand on the consultation and drugs, and leaving looking like I had contracted a rare tropical skin disease, I felt lighter, less stressed. It felt good to be doing something instead of waiting and hoping for the best.

Maybe this natural/alternative treatment is the way to go.

TAG-TEAM OF LOVE

We had some of the guys here for dinner last night and laughed a lot. Brilliant evening. Because Mike and I, when we entertain, are always swapping and juggling and passing things to each other, Msibi calls us 'The Tag-Team of Love.'

...

Blakeway responded to my email. She recommends surgery and wishes me luck.

WOMBS WITH A VIEW

Both Mandie and Roela have offered to be surrogates for us. How amazing are these people who surround us? Of course, we are nowhere close to going the surrogate route yet, if ever, but how many people do you know who would let you borrow their womb, rent-free, for nine months? Who would go through morning sickness and endless doctors' visits and weight gain and stretch marks and bad eyesight, pimples, spider veins, maternity jeans and BIRTH out of pure human kindness? I'm gobsmacked and humbled by their generosity. I laughed out loud after each offer, saying I hoped it wouldn't come to that, and Thank You Very Much, as if I were all of a sudden an awkward English aristocrat who had been offered the last cream scone that I had been dying to eat.

HAVE MORE SEX

As part of my *Positive Thinking!* and natural remedies and general attempt to avoid surgery and get pregnant with as little intervention as possible, I have embraced my inner hippie and done the following:

1. Scoured all the magazines in the house for pictures of pregnant bellies, beautiful babies and nursery ideas (impossibly soft bunnies with extra-large ears) — things so cute that my ovaries almost broke into song. I made a collage, which I've put up in my office (and of course hide whenever someone comes to visit — can't stand the imagined pity in their eyes. An infertile woman spending hours making a collage of babies and then staring at it every day. OMG, how very sad on so many levels). When I look at it I actually feel more hope than sadness.

2. I bought a fertility hypnotherapy track online and have it on my phone. I try to listen to it as often as possible. It's lovely — full of little acorn-grubbing squirrels and scampering baby animals and warm breezes and trees and birds that whisper. It makes me feel less like a barren mess and more like an amateur Mother Nature who just needs a little help to get the fecundity going.

3. No more hot baths and no more going to the steam room after gym - I read that the high temp is bad for

fertility.

4. My current yoga classes — 3 times a week —
will from now on be extra mindful and dedicated to my
much maligned uterus. Instead of planning my next novel /
worrying about late shipments and urgent orders /
thinking about sex, I will think Happy Uterus thoughts.

5. Have more sex. One of the extremely few upsides
to this, ahem, position, we find ourselves in, is that we get
to get lucky more often. I'm going to be 'O'-ing all over the
place. In the car, in the coffee shop, in the Woolworths
frozen food aisle. That's ovulating, to you.

6. Take my temperature every morning as per
Blakeway's ovulation chart, so that I can make sure we are
doing the dirty at the right time and not missing my
ovulation window. So much for 'not trying' — can't believe
I ever thought we should 'not try'.

7. Put a pillow under my bum after doing it, to
make sure the swimmers stay in the dedicated swimmers'
area.

8. Schedule regular acupuncture and reflexology
sessions.

9. Take my Chinese meds, plus a base (alkaline)
powder to combat the acidity in my body.

10. No more shooters, Red Bull or binge-drinking.
Now that I'm not in advertising anymore and Mike has
given up drinking, I don't (often) party like that anyway.

11. But don't even think of prying that occasional

reasonably-sized glass of wine / cold bottle of beer from my hands.

12. No more everyday coffee or ceylon. Can have occasionally as above.

13. Everything in moderation — including moderation.

14. No more getting up at 5am every morning to run 8km. Surprisingly, this is proving to be easier to give up than coffee.

So much for 'Not Trying'.

THE KILLERS

We went to see The Killers – they were excellent on stage. I felt hot-blooded; hopped up on painkillers and that terrible watery beer they sell in plastic beakers. You have to buy two or three at a time so that you don't miss the concert, but then they're a nuisance to hold and get warm so quickly, so you end up gulping them down like a 15-year-old at a high school social.

So there I was, high on everything but life and then the music starting whipping up my emotions. I felt such a connection to the band that it felt like they were singing to me. The lights and the sound and being with friends who were dancing their pants off. The lyrics made sense to me, comforted me. I got that clean hit of colour in my head, like when I meditate drunk.

'Everything is going to be alright.'

This has happened to me before. When I'm very happy or very sad, things talk to me. Things shimmer. It happens a lot when I travel, especially when I'm alone. On a bad day a few months ago, I stopped at a stop sign on a quiet road, and a little bird flew down and perched on the sign, as if it was looking at me. As if it was sent from somewhere. And a knowledge rushes at me and fills my heart, that indeed, everything IS going to be okay.

We Won't Do IVF

My eyes wander over my scribbles and I see 'IVF' 'IVF' 'IVF' everywhere. A year ago, smug in my ignorance of my fertility problems, I would never have considered it. I can recall whisky-fuelled conversations with close friends on the topic where I was the one leading the debate against it. Not as a therapy - I have nothing against it as a therapy, in fact I think it is pretty amazing — but as a therapy in the context of the situation in South Africa, where there are millions of orphans. Little souls desperate for love and nurturing, and here I am, desperate to love and nurture.

Mike and I have agreed that we will not do IVF. How could we?

8

THAT'S IT, I'M CRACKERS

I've decided I need to see a shrink. I need help to process this shitstorm that is my stuttering babymaker.

Mike and I used to have this amazing 'therapist': she was a crazy kind of numerologist-slash-Jungian-analyst. She used to sit and listen to you and smoke menthol cigarettes. At first you think she is some kind of quack, but then she surprises you with a little nugget of wisdom that you put in your brain-pocket to keep forever.

She was like Ramtha, but without the creepy possessed-by-a-ghost thing. She would talk in widening circles of wisdom, dropping ideas like little wrapped sweets around her. You gathered what was relevant to you. A chain-smoking oracle. She used to facilitate a kind of self-awareness workshop where she gently interrogated you and the other people in the room. It was interesting and a bit scary.

So it turns out that now, when I really do need a therapist, she's in New Zealand.

A friend recommended someone she had seen a while ago. She is really more of a relationship counsellor than a Crackers Counsellor but she isn't too far from here and I think I'll give her a go. Besides, her name is Micky. Who wouldn't want a shrink called Micky? I wonder how many times her husband has heard the line 'Are you taking the Micky?'

Or maybe she doesn't have a husband. Maybe she's good at listening but really terrible at relationships. Or the other way around. I guess there's only one way to find out.

If she is terrible, at least it will make a good story.

WHAT LOVELY CHICKEN

I cried in a restaurant. Mike's father, Chris, a debonair divorcé, took Mike and I out for dinner. We were discussing my faulty baby cannon. I was saying that maybe we should start some kind of fertility treatment but Mike doesn't want to. I don't blame him — I don't WANT to, either, but I want a baby more than I don't want treatment. I felt my throat close, so excused myself to have a little cry in the restroom. I scolded myself in the mirror, told myself not to be such a bloody drama queen, to put on my big girl panties and deal. But the tears came, anyway.

Chris was kind about pretending not to notice my smudged eyes when I came back to the table. Or maybe he really didn't notice. The boys are always teasing him for not being particularly observant. They tell the story of when they were all younger and sitting around after a family dinner, and Chris saying 'What lovely chicken!' and they would all crack up, laughing and holding their tummies. This happened regularly. The meal had, of course, been fish.

9

IVF IS FOR MONSTERS

I am picturing the orphaned babies, born lonely. I imagine that they are cold and I want to cry.

And then I think of IVF and my empty, sad sack of a uterus, and wonder how on earth I could ever consider such a horrible and selfish thing.

THE MEMORY OF WATER

Mandie, Avish and Mike took me out for a celebratory lunch: I have finished my second novel, 'The Memory of Water'. I started it in 2008 and it took me two years of stolen moments to finish.

I learnt from my writing mentor, Mister L, that you shouldn't wait for the publishing contract to celebrate. He always pops a bottle of the good stuff when he finishes writing his last page. Publishing contracts in South Africa are hard to come by, usually not worth much, and are not always based on merit. Publishing should be seen as a bonus, and nothing else. And so we celebrated. It was great to think about something else. It was a lovely afternoon, sitting at an outside table by a river with the guys and drinking chardonnay. The sense of accomplishment felt good. At least with my writing, if I put the hours in, I know that I will end up with something.

Okay, So Maybe IVF Isn't That Bad

I know, I know, I'm a hypocrite. Consider me slicked in an appropriate amount of hot self-loathing.

A few things have happened to bring me round to this massive U-turn of my moral compass.

1. My best friend from high school, who is living in the UK, has been battling to fall pregnant. Her doc has advised them that there is no way they'll fall pregnant without ICSI IVF. Pin is quite possibly the nicest human being in the world, and would make the best mother. We all now know that fertility has nothing to do with merit, but really, if anyone deserves to be a mom it is her. They're going to go ahead with IVF.

2. Who the fuck am I to judge that decision?

3. And it therefore follows that if I am not going to judge them, why should I judge myself? Surely my scathing disapproval should be consistently applied?

Look, to be honest, it's not that convenient. It's not

like I woke up and pulled on my 'I <3 IVF' shirt. The idea still makes me feel intensely uncomfortable. But for the first time today, I am allowing myself to consider, just consider, the idea of IVF, if, and only if, all else fails.

It makes me feel less hopeless, knowing that out there in the scary sci-fi world of test-tube babies, there may be a solution for us. It's like someone has laid out a nice soft safety net just in case I am driven to jump. I hope that it doesn't come to that. At this point in my life I don't have the energy to deal with so much cognitive dissonance. I'd be walking around, jangling, like some giant red tambourine. Also, I'm a bookseller and a writer, for fuck's sake, I don't have 50,000 rand to gamble.

...

Pin has started her IVF cycle. I think about her every day. She's worried that it won't work. I told her it would. It had better bloody work! It's hard being so far away from her. I wish I could support her more. I am fascinated by the process and ask her all the details. I dedicate my yoga practices to her and her precious little embryo. 'Stick, little embryo, stick!' I think at night while I lie in bed thinking of them. 'If you know what is good for you, you'll stick around.' If I was a soul floating around, weighing up my options, looking to start a new human life from scratch, Pin's is the uterus I'd choose.

10

U N - K N I T T E D

It's been 10 months since I binned the blister pack that used to contain my pill. The BFG wants me to go for some tests.

'So, about your devil womb,' he said in his Dutch accent (but not in so many words), 'it's freaky and we're going to need to check it out.' Okay, he didn't really say that.

'Because you have a scary-as-shit double-horn, we need to make sure that you don't have weirdo double-anything-else, you organ-doppelgänger.' He didn't say that either, but you get the idea.

The bicorniate uterus scenario is a congenital thing: it happens while you are a developing foetus. Usually when you need two of something (like lungs) your cells form things that split *et voila!* One becomes two. Sometimes it works the other way around, and two things will merge to form one. As with any stage of development, if there is some kind of genetic accident, or a biological glitch, things can go wrong. In my case, the BFG says that the pair of things meant to knit together to form my uterus only got 60% of the job done, hence the top of my uterus being ... un-knitted. Only halfway zipped. The case being such, who knows what else was melded / not melded enough / doubled up like cheap gin on a discount cruise? We'll need to have a proper look-see.

11

THEY START TYING HER DOWN

Oh my *hat* that was the worst experience ever.

It was like being in a medically-themed horror movie. You know the ones. Rusty equipment, maniacal doctors, needles the size of toothpicks. It was terrifying.

Picture this: Open on young fresh-faced girl (in jeans and a cheap and cheerful cereal-themed shirt from Thailand) showing up at a nice-enough hospital. Waiting and waiting and filling out reams of medical forms, while thinking of the work she is missing: she runs her own business and every lost hour counts. She thinks of the emails bottlenecking in her inbox, the deliverymen of urgent orders ringing the doorbell of her empty house. She is then presented with the estimated costs of the procedures she is to undergo and almost faints. She doesn't know if her medical aid will cover it, as it relates to infertility and medical aids are UncleFuckers when it comes to that, even though infertility is a disease recognised by the WHO.

Eventually she is given a backless hospital gown the colour of well-chewed gum and told to strip. She isn't allowed to wear undies, or her engagement ring. She's taken to a room where she lies on a cold stainless steel table, next to a tray holding a giant syringe on a hospital-blue napkin. Above her is a huge X-ray machine that looks a hundred years old. Despite the metal table leaching the warmth from her back and making it ache, she starts perspiring. They start tying her down.

'The restraints are so that you don't move while the machine is taking pictures,' says the smiley young nurse.

The radiologist walks in, wearing a curt expression and her customary radiation-proof armour.

'We're going to inject you with iodine,' she says, as if that is a perfectly polite thing to do. 'The X-ray will pick up the iodine in your bloodstream and show us its passage – show us your renal system – to see if there is a problem there.'

The BFG had explained that the biggest concern is that I have either only one kidney, or two sets of two. Four kidneys, I reckoned, was a bonus. No wonder I could keep up with drinking beer with the boys. Four kidneys! Maybe I could sell some to pay for this X-ray. One kidney, on the other hand, would not be so lucky. How funny that I just assumed that I had two to begin with. Brainwashed by biology lessons. How many do I really have? Bets, anyone? It could be like a game, if this room wasn't so damn scary.

After the iodine is pushed into the sweat-soaked girl's body, the horror film takes on a comedic slant, as all good/bad horror movies do. To work the ancient machine, the nurse has to run from one side of the room to the other, dragging the heavy ceiling-mounted contraption along with her while it shudders on its rails, threatening to fall off and crush all three of the people beneath it. Bang! Bang! Bang! Bang! it goes on every passage. Underneath the banging is a whirring, a clicking, as the X-ray film is exposed.

'Again,' says the radiologist. Again, again, again. Banging and clicking and whirring until the nurse is out of breath from running and dragging and still the radiologist wants more, adjusting my pose in between.

'Again,' she says, relentless, some kind of insane perfectionist.

'These pictures aren't for the fucking World Press Photo awards,' the patient doesn't say out loud. She looks at the other women in the room, protected by their heavy aprons. Thinks that this large dose of radiation can't be good for her organs, either. What does a radiologist know about fertility? And with fertility at stake, who cares, anyway, about an extra kidney either way? She imagines the rays bombarding her ovaries, zapping her eggs by the thousands. Microwaving her babymaker. Wouldn't it be terrible, she thinks, if the very first procedure she undergoes in order to get pregnant actually renders her forever infertile? She sweats some more.

STRANGER THINGS HAVE HAPPENED

The radiologist's report gave me the all-clear. No double renal system, no bonus kidneys. The BFG told me that in really rare cases women can have ENTIRE DOUBLE BABYMAKERS. That's two of absolutely everything, including vajayjays. I told a male friend this and he looked really interested. I was like, 'Right?' (thinking it was fascinating) and he was, like, 'Right,' (thinking of the pornographic possibilities). I was shocked. The sexual side of it didn't even cross my mind. Did. Not. Occur.

It's official, then. The horny person I used to be has been replaced by a crazy, frustrated, broken baby-making machine. I wanted to throw myself onto the ground and wail. Instead, we drank vast quantities of whisky. Where are those extra kidneys when you need them? I still have a headache. Thank God for friends.

12

No More Fresh Heartbreak

Driving home from a particularly difficult session with Micky today — we agreed that if by some miracle I do manage to conceive, knowing that my chances of miscarriage are so high, it would be best to wait until the last trimester to start buying baby things and decorate the nursery — I got a call from an international number. Knowing it could only be either a call centre in India peddling Facebook advertising or my precious Pin, I almost mounted a pavement in my rush to stop the car and answer. She told me her test came back positive. POSITIVE! She is pregnant! Her IVF worked. She is pregnant pregnant pregnant! My face melted. Such relief. She wouldn't have to deal with any more procedures. No more (fertility) disappointments, no more fresh heartbreak. After we ended the call I sat in my car and wept.

I SPOKE MONKEY

In the effort to be more Zen we, along with our closest friends Mandie and Avish, decided to go to the meditation course at the Nan Hua buddhist temple in Bronkhorstspruit. Huge bling building in the middle of nowhere. Vegetarian chinese noodles for breakfast, lunch and dinner. No alcohol allowed - which of course made me want to smuggle in some miniature bottles of vodka. Also: no sex. No co-ed bunking, whether you're married or not. I know what you're thinking: it would be difficult to get pregnant in a place like that.

They taught us different ways to meditate, which was cool. You know there's the old-school sitting in lotus position and that's what you think of when you think of meditation, but we did a meditation to music, a walking meditation, and a tea meditation.

I liked them all, and the tea meditation was lovely. They showed us how to make a small pot of green tea, doing it so that you are completely and utterly present in the moment. The lesson was simple: almost any of your everyday tasks can be a meditation, as long as you are able to empty your mind. You could switch on the kettle and think a thousand things and before you realise it you have not only made yourself tea but also tipped it down your throat, hardly tasting it. Or you could take the time to stand there, breathe, empty your mind of unnecessary thoughts (most are unnecessary), hear the water warm up and boil, and slowly and thoughtfully make your tea. You have not lost anything by taking the extra time, to the contrary, you have gained a mindful experience, and you can move on to your next task refreshed.

In the end it's all about being in the moment. You could be having sex and meditating at the same time (okay, they didn't say this, *per se*, but it makes sense — I am probably more 'in the moment' during sex than when doing anything else). Yoga, running, walking and gardening, for me, are other ways of meditating, I just never realised it.

I know I think too much. Always have. It's not like I'm an intellectual or anything, I'm just too self-aware for my own good. I play things over in my mind until they are sufficiently processed, and only then can I let go. Even a casual conversation for me is hard work. It's angst-y. Small talk, more so. It's like there is the actual conversation taking place in real time, and then there is the echo further back in my head, analysing everything I say and how it could be incorrectly interpreted.

I like spending time on my own, I crave it, but I am not always easy company.

This blip, this hesitation to talk, has always been with me: I've been like this since I can remember. My mother always tells the story of when I started talking as a toddler; it was years late by regular milestone standards.

I was so quiet that once my parents forgot — literally FORGOT — me at our holiday accommodation while they trundled off to the beach. They got as far as unpacking the buckets and spades before realising something was amiss, or, rather, that someone was missing.

'Here's Neets's towel,' my mom always says when she tells the story, using her hands to unpack the invisible beach bag. 'Here's Neets's — er, hang on. Where's Neets?'

In their defence, I was huddled up against a cool wall, under my bed, so engrossed in a book that I didn't even realise that they had left. I was easy to miss.

When I wasn't haunting holiday beds with my mute-like, stringy-haired countenance, that is to say: when I wasn't quiet, I was speaking Monkey. I spoke Monkey for ages (my older brother used to translate my grunting and gesturing) and the pressure to talk began to mount. My hearing was tested. I was coaxed by strangers with soggy biscuits. I remember feeling anxious to speak because my lack-lustre lexicon had become A Thing. I'm sure I would have chatted sooner if it wasn't for everyone making such a big deal about it. Then one day, while we were on holiday at the South Coast we were all in the car and the pressure was off: no one had mentioned it for a while. I thought: I'm going to talk now. It was a decision. Instead of testing the water with a word or two, I said out loud: 'Oh, we had such a nice day at the beach today.' My father slammed on the brakes, almost crashed the car, thinking that they had taken the wrong child home.

Oh My God Shoot Me Now

Am I the only one who yells for my imaginary shotgun when I get an invitation to a baby shower?

I used to love the idea of them: a whole party dedicated to talking about babies and tiny clothes and gory stories of birth and breastfeeding. And you get to eat snacks, almost always including cupcakes. It's all about rallying together in support and generosity of spirit.

Seriously, who could hate that? Only the most miserable of humans, surely, only very-smelly cave-dwelling pond-scum.

But if I am honest, really honest, I'd rather be anywhere else. I didn't enjoy them when I thought I was fertile, and I can't stand them now. The oestrogen-fueled gaggle, the baby-talk (*Shamepies! Ag jirre!* Look at those little sockies! Nunus!), the overly-sweet cakes, the stupid games (OMG the stupid games OMG) and the desperate lack of alcohol all add up to a very special kind of torture, made complete with comments like 'Just stop thinking about it and it will happen' and 'Just drink a bottle of tequila — that's what worked for us!'

I grin and bear it. After all, I keep reminding myself, it is about the pregnant friend, not about me. I try to not let the adorable onesie I buy upset me. The one with fat, dimpled, baby dinosaur print, matching leggings and hat. I try to not inhale the baby-powder scent of the packet of disposable nappies. I try to get in and out of Baby City as fast as my legs will take me, pretending I have somewhere better to be.

13

DARLING, WHAT ARE YOU DOING WITH THAT BUTCHER KNIFE

My shoulder is killing me.

The BFG gave me a script for stronger painkillers, but it's like the endo knows the medication has been upped and retaliates in kind. It's like a tentacled monster growing inside me, under my skin, invading my flesh, wrapping around my muscles. Pulling and squeezing and burning me. It's hard to act normal, difficult to do day-to-day things like shower and wash my hair. Mike gets home, hugs me, and asks if I have any ideas for dinner.

Dinner? I think.

I am living in some kind of parallel universe of pain where nothing matters except my next pill. Other people, normal people, are talking about dinner. About avo and haloumi wraps, spaghetti arrabiata, bangers and mash.

I open the cutlery drawer and see the butcher knife. I hold it up to him, glinting. I want to say: 'Please, cut it off. Cut my arm off.'

Instead, I start chopping onions.

...

I've always been relatively healthy. I almost wrote 'I've always been healthy' but that's because I forgot for a moment about what a sickly child I was. I don't remember much of it, but I had chronic asthma. I had my first attack as a baby — I turned blue — and my poor parents had to rush me to hospital, thinking their kid was dying. After that the attacks came regularly and my mom would just shoot me over to casualty and stick a big green nose (nebuliser) over my face while we waited to see a doctor. So this isn't the first time my body has let me down, but it feels like it is. It could be worse (it could always be worse), my mother would remind herself, sitting in the paediatric ward for one of those extended stays. She would look around at the other beds and pat her lips and whisper through the oxygen tent to me: It Could Be Worse.

KICK ME

You know what I hate? Up until my diagnosis, not a lot. Maybe just a little list. Animal cruelty. Bigotry. Maggots. Mosquitoes. Margarine. Soggy cereal. The usual suspects.

But since I can't get pregnant? A list as long as a table at the Oktoberfest. But here I'll keep it fertility-related, or we could be here all day.

I hate it when people tell me how easy it was for them to conceive.

'All your father had to do was sneeze and I was pregnant' (from the one mom).

'Your father hung his underpants on the line and bam! I was pregnant' (from the other).

'We never thought much about it in those days,' says one of the dads. 'It just kind of happened.'

'Thanks guys,' I don't say. 'That sure makes me feel better about the whole thing.'

I hate it when people say things like 'It will happen when it's meant to happen' (I used to think this. It is a silly thing to think). It would make no sense to apply it to anything else, so why fertility?

I also hate it when people give advice. Have you tried homeopathy / meditation / SCIO machine / this doctor / that doctor / this diet / cutting out alcohol / cutting out caffeine / having your auras cleansed / having sex on your head / etc.? It worked for this person my aunt's tenant's mistress knows. You know what also works? ADOPTION.

'Just adopt,' they say. 'Then you'll get pregnant immediately. It happened to so-and-so's so-and-so.'

I sigh and facepalm. JC on a cracker, what am I working with here?

Above all, *above all*, I hate it when people hint at the idea that if I just 'relax' it will happen.

'Really?!' I want to scream (to prove how very un-fucking-relaxed I can be). I have a devil uterus and a messy spider web of endometriosis tangling up my tubes. You really think putting my feet up every now and then is going to cure that?

Structural womb-issues aside, endometriosis is a disease. Terrorist cells are invading my insides and taking my pipework and my dreams hostage. It's like a non-fatal form of cancer. Would you tell someone with cancer to 'relax'? Would you advise someone with diabetes to 'just go on an island holiday cruise'?

14

The Crackers Counsellor

In March 2010 I met my Crackers Counsellor. I resisted the urge to sing: 'Hey Micky, you're so fine, you're so fine you-blow-my-mind!' mostly because I was drizzing for 50 minutes of the hour.

Look, she's human. She was a bit taken aback by the story and the accompanying waterworks. She looked at me with real concern and I could see her thinking: 'This chick is fucked.' Or, maybe: 'Hopeless! You poor girl, you don't need a psychologist, you need a shiny new babymaker.'

She said I needed to express my feelings often and without reserve, in order to process the constant bad news. Infertility is not a once-off trauma that you slowly get over. Rather, it hurts you every month (in my case, literally and emotionally), and when you are stuck in that cycle it's difficult to have perspective and to heal. I told her I have this journal, for that reason. I'm sure no one I know wants to hear about the ins and outs of my designer uterus. I've always been more of a writer than a talker, anyway.

...

One of the reasons I don't like the idea of fertility treatments is that it feels like we are trying to force an outcome. In my experience, trying to force something does not often work. My mom used to say to us as kids 'Don't force it!' when we were trying to bludgeon something or other into working. If you force it you can break it.

Usually I find that if things fall into place easily, it can be taken as a sign that you are heading in the right direction. I used to be quite sure of this philosophy.

But.

I am meant to be a mother. Nothing in my life is truer than that. That truth runs deep, it's set in my bones. So here is one of the (many) lessons infertility has taught me: don't be too sure of anything.

THINGS I AM GRATEFUL FOR

It strikes me how bloody ungrateful I am for everything I have.

Sometimes when I see people begging with sunburnt toddlers strapped to their backs on main road islands, or the fifth feather-duster man of the week, I think what a wastrel I am. I have so much, how can I possibly justify being this sad?

What really brought it home was seeing Mike's dad

the other night (he lives a few of roads up from our house so we see each other all the time). Chris was diagnosed with terminal cancer a couple of years ago but you'd never guess it from looking at him. He is on round after round of chemo but he never complains about so much as a headache. He knows the Multiple Myeloma (blood/bone cancer on the spectrum between Leukemia and Lymphoma) will make him very sick eventually (he was given 3 or 4 years to live), so he is living as much as he can now. His way and his spirit makes it easy to forget that he has cancer. You see him, panama hat on, driving his SL with the top down, on the way to fetch a newspaper and a takeaway cappuccino, or to have lunch with one of his lady friends, and you'd never guess that he's terminal.

He can see when I am in pain just by looking at my face, and is always sympathetic. It makes me feel like such a *doos*. Here I am feeling sorry for myself and my sore shoulder, wanting to just climb into bed and wish the world away, while he is upbeat and optimistic and, surprise!, here to take us out for dinner.

I've heard often that a good way to combat depression (or to just be happier) is to keep a gratitude journal. While I find that idea twee, I thought I'd just stop being such a grinch and write a bloody list. As you may have gathered, I like lists. And even grinches have things they are grateful for, like puppies to scare and little children to disappoint.

THINGS I AM GRATEFUL FOR:

1. My family. Mike's family. Our friends.

2. Mike. What's not to be grateful for? Intelligent, kind, funny (funny ha-ha, not funny-looking), in fact, incredibly good looking, sexy, etc. Sure he has faults (thank goodness) but it wouldn't be in the spirit of this list to point them out.

3. Our cats, Alex and Cocoa. They are my surrogate babies.

4. My business. I love my job, and I love being self-employed. Sure, I'm chained to my desk 24/7, but at least I'm doing something I love. I get to talk about, read about, and order books all day long.

5. My writing. I would hate to not write. After having written, the world just seems like a better place. Writing is my happy place.

6. My house. I love living in Parkhurst and being able to stroll up the road for dinner.

7. My garden, specifically the old-fashioned plants the previous owner left us with: Boston Ivy, vintage-looking irises, rhubarb.

8. My legs. Not because they're good legs (okay, maybe a little), but because I have two of them and they work. I love walking and running and yoga, which would be difficult to do without legs.

9. Okay, I'm running out of things here. Ah — I am

grateful for lists. They allow me to feel like I have some small measure of control over my life. They are calming. They stop the world from becoming overwhelming.

      10. Wait, have I said 'WINE'? Wine. There, that's ten.

15

THE DRUGS DON'T WORK

When people asked me to explain what endometriosis is, I'd go through the whole *spiel:* the rogue endometrial cells, the adhesions, the tangled babymaker bits. When I got bored of that (no one really seemed to know what I was talking about anyway, and seemed to want to redirect the conversation), I started telling a simplified version: My insides have been sewn together by evil stitches and it hurts to breathe. Sometimes its strings try to pull me to the floor, like a reverse puppet.

Now my explanation is even simpler. I just tell them that my uterus is trying to kill me.

...

Last night I couldn't sleep - the knife in my shoulder decided it was restless and that it wanted to do a little travelling. It slashed the top of my arm, dug a bit at my collarbone, then lodged itself snugly into my ribs. It felt like I was being beaten up from the inside. The top right quadrant of my body is being haunted by (a presumably shy) Jack the Ripper.

When this happens, breathing is agony. Crying makes it worse but I can't help it. I sit upright, hot tears on my cheeks, trying to breathe as shallowly as possible. Mind is a fog - lost in the messy pain.

I took double the amount of Myprodol, then triple. I mixed it up with Nurofen. At 3am when I couldn't take the stabbing anymore I hunted for a sleeping pill, knowing it was a bad idea, but didn't find one. After upending the medicine box on the bathroom floor I sat there, hot shoulder on cold bath tiles, counting the painkillers I had left and the hours it would take until the sun came up.

Mike tries to comfort me — he knows not to touch me on fear of incineration — but doesn't know what to say. What is there to say? When I feel like this the only person I want to see is a medically-trained field soldier. The guys in war movies who bite off the cap of the morphine injection before punching it into your thigh. It's a fantasy I replay in my head. Camo gear, shoe-polished cheeks, kind eyes made watery by the smoke of gunblasts and bombs. A grey bashed-up tin case full of opiates ready to be injected directly into my bloodstream. My dream man. More intimate than sex: I want to open my veins to him. This is my fantasy now. How life changes. How life changes you.

This morning I know the attack is over. I feel bruised inside, my ribs feel broken, but the active stabbing is over. The heat is gone, replaced by an ebbing ache. I wonder what damage this episode has done to my insides. I know that my body, with its best intentions, will try to paper over the damage: covering the misplaced endometrial cells with scar tissue. And next month, those cells will re-swell, tearing the new tissue apart. These layers upon layers of scar tissue and rogue cells are in the process of forming sticky strings, called adhesions, which can glue organs together, and other mischief. I picture these pieces of pink sticky-tape radiating off my diaphragm like paper streamers from a fan, reaching for my lungs and liver. I wonder what other pieces of me are already stuck together, and if that is one of the reasons I am not yet pregnant.

The BFG says that I don't necessarily have pelvic endometriosis. To the contrary, he reasons, I don't have any of the pelvic endo symptoms.

Yes, it would be good to know for sure, but this involves surgery — a laparoscopy — and is not to be done on a whim. Under general anaesthetic, four incisions are made in your abdomen. Through these cuts the surgeon is able to see, via a scope, what state your insides are in. He can also, if he finds endo, get rid of it, and in so doing, untangle what needs untangling.

As much as my babymaker is concerning me, at the moment I need to know what can be done about my diaphragm. It is as simple as this: I can't live with this intense pain. And I can't live with knowing that it is coming back next month, and then the next month. The idea fills me with an anxiety I have never felt before. I can't do it and I don't know what to do about it.

The BFG says they can operate on diaphragmatic endo, but it's not as simple as a laparoscopy. Diaphragmatic endometriosis calls for its big brother, a laparotomy, where they slice you from breastbone to bikini line. When I go pale as he describes the surgery, he tries to cheer me up. Of course, he says, the preferred treatment is pregnancy! Pregnancy cures endo of all forms for the duration of the pregnancy, sometimes indefinitely.

But, wait, endo causes infertility. Oh, the irony. Ha.

I feel like I am missing something important (and by that I don't mean a decent uterus, although that also seems to be the case). I feel like I am in a children's story that doesn't make sense. A farcical Black-Adderesque tale. I am the poor little girl dressed in rags whose fairy godmother visits to grant her a wish. The grubby (but kind-hearted) girl tells her that more than anything, she'd like a kitten. The FG waves her wand and says 'You may have your kitten. Of course! But first you must get a kitten.'

The little girl doesn't understand. 'But the reason I am asking for your help is because I can't find a kitten anywhere. I've looked and looked and there are no kittens to be found.'

'Don't you see?' demands the stupid FG, 'once you find the kitten then you'll have a kitten!'

So we have to make the choice between a fish-gutting surgery or an indefinite wait to (miraculously) get knocked up, with the pain getting worse every month. Of course, there is also the option of going back on the pill and forgetting about having children altogether, but that would just cause a different pain. Being a hippie that is scared of surgery, I think we will try for a few more months and then re-assess the impossible situation.

For now, I need stronger drugs, even if it means buying them from the back of a petrol station in Hillbrow. I'm sorry Mr Drugdealer — you say you're out of stock, that you only have horse tranquillisers? Bring it! I'm in.

Rohypnol all of a sudden has a lovely ring to it. Maybe Mike will roofie me, if I ask him nicely.

...

A few weeks ago my GP, bless him, gave me a script for a schedule 5 drug that's illegal in some countries. Apparently it can be 'deadly'. I don't care. It works like a bomb.

The anxiety that builds when I start to feel any glimmer of pain — knowing how bad it's going to get — and when it catches me off-guard: the panic of realising that I don't have my painkillers with me. The other day I was driving home to my drugs and hit traffic. I was already very uncomfortable and knew that the extra 15 minutes it would take me to get home would hurt a lot. I began sweating, my heart was battering itself against my breastbone. There was noise in my head — I had to speak loudly to myself to be heard — saying that it would be okay, it was just pain. It was just pain. There are also the times that I take the drugs before going out to dinner and leave the rest of them at home on purpose so that I'm not tempted to overdose. Usually it works out okay, but sometimes it starts hurting before we leave and then even though we make a quick exit I am weeping on the drive home.

It's not those times that make me think I need to be careful with addiction - it's the times that I'm not in pain but find myself thinking about the pills. They are not cravings, not exactly, but wandering thoughts that attach to my shoulder, like a cartoon devil, and nag for a while.

If I feel that I am likely to overdose I give Mike my pills: he knows to dispense them only after a certain amount of time (2 tabs every 6–8 hours). Sometimes he is strict with it, other times he knows better. Sometimes I bargain with him.

Me: 'I need more.'

Him: 'No.'

WTF? Who does he think he is, a fucking prison warden?

Him: 'It's only been 4 hours since the last 2.'

Me: 'I know, but 4 hours is almost 6 hours.'

(He gives me a paternal disappointed/annoyed look.)

Me: 'How about if I take 1 more now, then I'll only take another 1 in 2 hours.'

Him: 'You know that's not true, so, no.'

Me: 'Okay, half now, 1 and a half in 2 hours.'

Him: 'Half isn't going to do anything.'

Me: (start crying)

Him: (hands over pills)

...

The pain today is unbearable. I can't think straight. I had to give my pills to Mike because I thought if I didn't I would just lose it and take them all in one go. Schedule 5 and they don't even work properly. They are like fucking band-aids for a broken arm. I'm in so much pain. I can't do this anymore. I don't want to live like this. I fucking hate my life.

...

Think of Grumpy Cat. Now think of my uterus. Now think of Grumpy Cat again. What? You can't notice a difference? Me neither.

16

LET LOVE RUST

It is our first wedding anniversary today.

It's not something I want to celebrate. After all, it means that we have been trying to fall pregnant for a year with no success. 12 failed cycles. 12 times I have hoped and been disappointed. Worse than the disappointment: the physical pain. Yes, there is emotional pain, like a smooth cold stone in my heart, but it is less invasive than the knife in my shoulder.

We are now officially/clinically/medically 'infertile'. The upside: now that it is official, it becomes a problem to be solved.

Another upside: Maybe now people will stop telling me that if I just 'relax' or 'stress less' we'd conceive, as if going on an island holiday and drinking mojitos would magically reform my wonky womb and re-stitch my diaphragm.

It's not that I'm not happy to be married to Mike. Despite my reservations about marriage I'm finding it good. I don't think it has changed the relationship much, which was one of my concerns — but maybe that comes later. The important thing to me is not that we've been married for a year, but that we've been together for eight years. Eight solid years of love, respect, affection. I don't believe in single soul-mates, but I can't imagine being with anyone else.

It's been a shit year, so it's hard to celebrate. How do you honour a year of bad luck? Should you? It would feel disingenuous to crack open a bottle of sparkly and have a dance. I don't want to celebrate. Unless we do it by sitting in a dim room, sighing 'Fuck It,' listening to blues, drinking too much whisky. I could do that. Or maybe the silver lining is that at least the year is over.

While I was completely avoiding the idea of the anniversary, Mike went to a lot of trouble finding the perfect anniversary gift. He commissioned Roela's husband, Flip, to make a notebook for us — to write letters to each other every year. It's hand-made and a bit messy — a bit like a good marriage, I guess — and beautiful. It has substance and texture. It feels good in my hands. I couldn't think of a more thoughtful present. I guess I should have been a little more thoughtful than giving him a scribbled letter and a Big Lebowski DVD.

Hey, no one said I would make a good wife.

17

Heart vs. Brain

I feel like my body has betrayed me in the worst way possible. My brain yells at my heart to not be so fucking sensitive.

'The worst way possible?' it screeches. 'Really?'

'Yes,' my heart says, 'and it fucking hurts!'

'Oh, grow a pair!' the brain yells.

'Of ovaries that work?' the heart shouts back. 'I'd love to!'

'So you're infertile, you think you're the first?'

'It feels like it. It's lonely.'

'Boo hoo. You're infertile. You're not the first. Deal with it.'

'Don't use that ugly word, I hate it. Sob!'

The brain sighs.

'Do you know what could be a worse betrayal than your precious babymaker?' it asks. 'That your eyes stop working. Or your mouth, or your legs.'

'Yes,' the heart says, 'you're right. That would be worse. Good point. That's probably why you're the brain.'

'So, actually, you should be grateful.'

'I wouldn't go that fucking far.'

18

MONSTER SPERM

So, yes, it's May 2010 and I've been taking prenatal folic acid religiously for a year now. 365 little pills. I may as well have built a medium-sized snowman out of them for all the use they were to me.

I went back to the BFG, this time dragging Mike along.

It didn't start well. His receptionist is a banshee from the third rung of hell. It's a quiet space, the waiting room, until she opens her infernal mouth.

'You here for a PAP SMEAR?' she demands.

I am sitting with Mike, leafing through a tattered copy of Elle, minding my own business. Everyone else in the waiting room stops what they are doing and looks at me.

Oh! I realise. She's speaking to me. Despite me not

being anywhere near the counter, and not being scheduled for a pap smear. She repeats her question. I hurry up to her and tell her why we're here, which she repeats loudly for all to hear.

It's not like I'm ashamed of my fertility issues. To the contrary, I'll tell whoever will listen about my medically-marvellous heart-shaped uterus. But this woman had no shame. I wanted to stuff her overly lipsticked mouth with a maternity pad. Poor Mike — of English descent, bless his sometimes-stiff upper lip — baulked. Confusion creased his brow; you could see him wondering if this was really happening. 'My dear lady,' I imagined him saying in a posh English accent, perhaps like Colin Farrell's Darcy, 'did you just shout out *pap smear?*'

I blushed and blushed. I'm a blusher. I blush when I'm embarrassed; when I'm shy; when I'm not embarrassed or shy; when I'm turned on, when more than one person looks at me at a time; when I am trying to get a point across and not managing it particularly well; when I (worst nightmare) speak in public. I have never tried to do all these things at the same time but I imagine that if I ever do I will explode all over everyone, leaving bits of myself on their coats and on the floor. The scarlet suicide bomber.

Sometimes the warm beginning of a blush embarrasses me, and then I go into full steaming red-face. If people remark on it, it gets even worse. I'm talking a hot-scalp crimson-ears blush, usually accompanied by perspiration. It's not pretty. Despite speaking in hushed tones to the demonic receptionist, to give her a clue that perhaps not all patients liked to have their vaginal health discussed at full volume in front of a roomful of strangers,

she carried on with her yelling. 'Are you PREG-NANT?'
she bellowed in her Afrikaans accent, despite me having
just told her, twice, that we were seeing the doctor to try to
GET PREGNANT. Her short red hair was styled to stand
up. It looked like hellfire.

The BFG was as lovely as always. He
recommended we do AI. That's artificial insemination, or
alien intelligence, depending on which movie you're
watching. It costs a tenth of the price of IVF. You usually
only consider it if there is a male factor issue.

Mike's SA (semen analysis) came in, and it was
surprising. He is a yogi who doesn't cycle, doesn't wear
tight undies, stays away from gluten and dairy, and doesn't
eat meat or drink alcohol.*.

*I know! I married a man who doesn't drink! Who
does that? But I fell in love with him when he was, shall we
say, less ascetic, and you know, love, man. What can you
do? He still has a beautiful soul.**

**At least, that's what I tell myself when I'm three
beers down and want to go dancing and he wants to go
home.

He has never smoked or been addicted to crack. So
I expected the results to arrive with a massive stamp of
approval, a giant emoticon of two thumbs up. Maybe a
bubble-sticker of a happy penis thrown in, for good
measure. But that wasn't the case.

While his overall count and mobility (the amount of
sperm per mil and the way they moved) was good, his

morphology was bad, at 7%. Morphology basically means the shape of the sperm. Only a regular-shaped tadpole can make the long, arduous journey to the egg. The other guys swim around happily in circles like drunk goldfish, and even if they were to reach the egg, they wouldn't be able to fertilise it. Of all of Mike's sperm, only 7% had a chance.

Of course the first thing I do is Google the numbers. After all, I kept thinking, 7% of a lot is good, isn't it? And he has a lot! At least it's better than 7% of a little bit. The interwebz had percentages and stats all over the place and they were difficult to make sense of, but on the WHO page I found exactly what I (wasn't) looking for. It said that anything below 15%, morphology-wise, was regarded as teratozoospermic, and in this case fertility treatment was recommended.

Finally, a word that is ugly enough to rival 'endometriosis'. Teratozoospermic, if you look at its Latin roots, means MONSTER SPERM. It would be funny, perhaps, in another context. If it wasn't happening to us. He could go to a Halloween party and not have to dress up. He could just gesture towards his nethers and say: 'I brought my MONSTER SPERM.'

In my head I imagine that receptionist shouting at us amid a particularly packed waiting room: 'Is this the one?' and when I look at her, askance, she'll shout louder: 'Is this the one with the MONSTER SPERM?'

In the shower, afterwards, trying to wash away what Google told me, I thought I might feel a little relieved. At least our problems falling pregnant were not *all* due to my malfunctioning babymaker. But I didn't, I don't.

If anything, it's the opposite of relief. It feels like one more problem to add to our toppling pile.

'Here!' booms the universe. 'Take this Teratozoospermicazoya-whatever and add it to your endometriosis and shapeshifter uterus.'

'Thanks,' I mumble, secretly giving him/her the finger.

The BFG recommended Mike take a supplement consisting of seven big red bullets a day. If that doesn't improve his, ahem, 'output,' then we can consider a hormone therapy drug that is also used to treat breast cancer. We don't like the sound of that, but if you spoke to us six months ago we'd tell you that we wouldn't do any fertility treatment. They lure you in slowly, these fertility doctors. First it's a few over-the-counter pills and next thing you're a guy on HRT. AI doesn't sound like such a big deal anymore, especially when you have IVF hovering on the horizon. What's a couple of injections and a turkey baster between friends? This is how they get you. What else can you do when you are being chased by monster sperm? You run down the (very slippery) slope.

...

So I was back at the hospital with the BFG today, in preparation for our turkey basting. Before we start with AI we need to make sure that my fallopian tubes are open. If they are blocked then there is obviously no way AI could work. Depending on their state, I may need surgery to open them. If that is not possible, the only remaining option would be IVF.

IVF circumvents the tubes completely as the eggs are harvested from the ovaries, fertilised, and then the embryos are transferred directly to the uterus. You'd think that IVF would have a higher success rate than 20 – 25% with all that help, but apparently implantation (the embryo burrowing into the uterine lining and staying there) is a very tricky issue, and there is very little anyone can do to influence whether it takes or not. The numbers in this game are too much of a gamble for my liking.

But, breathe, we are not there yet. As my friends tell me: Baby steps! (which now seems a slightly cruel thing to say).

The way to check if the tubes are open is to have an hysterosalpingogram test where you lie on a table with an x-ray machine above you and they slide a catheter up your vajayjay and into your uterus and fill it with a contrast dye. The dye then shows the shape of your uterus and, if your tubes are clear, it travels up along the two frilly lines far thinner and longer than you'd expect them to be. There is a screen in the room so you can watch it happen, which is quite cool. Picture a martini glass filling up with cola. It has twirly straws in it and the cola should travel up them, too. It's nerve-wracking stuff. I wouldn't have minded a cocktail just then.

Everyone seemed to hold their breath, waiting to see if the lines would appear or not. I had been warned that the dye can make you cramp, but I didn't feel anything but relief as my two dark scribbles appeared.

I felt a nonsensical pride in my body, lying on that stretcher. I ignored the smug heart-shape and thanked my babymaker for having wide open fallopian tubes. It had done something right, for a change.

SHOOTING UP IS NOT FOR SISSIES

The BFG taught Mike how to inject me. (Cue the stupid jokes — no wonder I wasn't getting pregnant if my husband didn't know how to inject me. He wasn't giving me the right shots. He didn't know what to do with his needle, etc.)

The stimming injection is to force my body to ovulate (even though I don't have a problem ovulating), and then the trigger shot ensures that the follicle releases the egg at exactly the right time.

Any number of things can and do go wrong.

For example, if your partner is rushing in the morning because he has an important client presentation to deliver, he may break the glass vial of saline while attempting to open it and cut open his finger, getting blood all over his work clothes. While he hunts for a plaster and a new set of clothes, you may try to suck up, from the kitchen table, any of the spilt saline you can see, and, finding there's not enough, wonder if you can top it up with water from the just-boiled kettle.

You may then not be able to get all the solution out of the second vial. You try again, only managing to pump more air bubbles into the syringe. You remember your brother telling you when you were sub-ten-years-old that if you inject an air bubble into someone's bloodstream they will die. You reason that a butt-cheek is very different to a main artery, but it makes you nervous nonetheless.

Finally, you may lower your knickers and lean over the kitchen table. Your partner, still in his underwear, not having found suitable replacement clothes, assumes his position behind you. He pushes it into you, ask you if it's in far enough. You swear at him — how are you supposed to know? And snap at him to get on with it. You look up to see that your domestic worker has walked into the room. You don't know how long she's been standing there. There is an awkward silence. Everyone is very late for work. Later, after the stinging in your bum has subsided, you see her scrubbing the table with bleach.

Precious Cargo

So we rock up at the sperm spinning place at the crack of dawn's bum, as requested. Why these things always have to start at 5 in the morning is beyond comprehension. We wait for a-a-a-a-ages to see someone. When it's Mike's turn to 'make his deposit' he's given a clear plastic tub and shown to a white room. I shuffle in behind him, awkwardly offering help, and am dismissed. Before I leave the room I see the one sad magazine in there to help things along. It's not pornographic, it's not even erotic, I think, as I page through it with dismay. It's just a few athletic-looking girls wearing bikinis. Not a brazilian or a nipple in sight. It makes me want to apologise to him. Next time I will be better prepared. I'll buy something new and bring it. A new thing every time. Lingerie, a magazine, a toy. It'll be fun. Or maybe there won't be a next time.

Maybe this will work. If the BFG is right and it is primarily a sperm issue, this AI could work.

It takes more than an hour for them to spin the sample, and then they give me the clean, new and improved, monster-reduced sperm. They tell me to keep it nestled in my cleavage, to keep it at body temperature. I don't stop them and say: 'Do you see any cleavage?' I just pop it into the middle of my bra and give it a little pat, the way I've seen people who keep cash there do. Precious cargo, I think.

We jump in the car and race to the BFG's rooms. You would swear I was nine and a half months' pregnant and in advanced labour the way we rushed there. When we get there we have to — of course — wait some more, while the doc is busy with another patient, perhaps performing a PAP SMEAR. We tap our feet and wring our hands and generally look as anxious as possible, hoping that we'll be bumped up the queue before any more of our soldiers bite the dust.

Eventually we are let in and the doc scans me. We see a big, ripe follicle, ready to burst. A perfect planet on the monochrome screen, surrounded by galaxies of stars. Our timing is excellent, he smiles: you're just about to ovulate. I decide I love his Dutch accent. Did you hear how beautiful that sounded? My ovaries are practically glowing from the compliment. He loads up the turkey-baster and does the deed while Mike holds my hand. If we can't conceive naturally, I think, at least we can say that we were holding hands when it happened.

My instinct is to lie down for as long as possible afterwards, to make sure that it stays in long enough to do its job, but after five minutes the doc kicks us out. We have to go back tomorrow for a top-up, just in case.

Turkey Baster Top-up

We went to a 80s party last night and danced in neon lights. Bright pink hoop earrings lie discarded in the cubby hole. The temptation after an AI is to go straight to bed and stay there, legs in the air, for as long as possible, but the science says that it doesn't alter the success rate.

The roads were cool and empty so early on a Sunday morning, decorated with some broken headlight glass and other Saturday night litter. We yawned in the car, smudged our eyes.

It was AI Groundhog Day for us: the same terribly tedious routine of waking up way too early to rush to wait, to rush to wait. A perfunctory orgasm in-between. A turkey-baster top-up.

This time it felt like the BFG took the baster out too early — when I stood up I felt it dribble down my thighs. I didn't mention it to Mike and tried not to think about it. I don't need an extra thing to worry about. Worry will not help me get pregnant.

We went to a café and had delicious, comforting food and talked about how it was possible that I would be pregnant in a few days' time. There was a lightness to the air around us. We were in a cocoon of optimism and tentative excitement. We let ourselves daydream about how our little baby will look (if we are lucky, the boy we both know it will be will have my hairline and Mike's hair, if not, the other way around, in which case we should start saving for infant hair plugs immediately), and played with baby names.

BETA-SCHMETA

After two weeks of wondering if every twinge and ache was pregnancy-related, I went for a blood test this morning. It's called a quantitative HCG. In the old days the test would just be a yes/no result, but this counts the HCG (pregnancy hormone), telling you how far along you are. That number is called your 'beta' and you pray for the largest number possible. A large number is comforting. A small number could mean anything from a 'missed' pregnancy (you were technically pregnant but it didn't stick) to a dangerous ectopic pregnancy (the embryo implanted into your fallopian tube). You could still have a healthy pregnancy with a low beta, as long it doubles every 48-ish hours.

The waiting in-between the drawing of the blood and the lab's phone call is torture. I tried to work to distract myself, but ended up staring at my screen, my heart rocketing out of my chest every time the phone rang. Of course today was the day that every colour-copier and insurance company decided to call me. I was polite to the first few.

The test came back negative. No popping non-alcoholic champers for me. I called Mike with the news — he wasn't surprised. I guess after a year of disappointments you come to expect bad news. The success rate of AI isn't high: only 8–15%, but our thinking was that's 8–15% higher than without it.

To rub salt in the wound, my shoulder started hurting this afternoon. I'm not sure why I paid for a blood test when I have an extremely reliable period-sensor built into my arm. Please pass the painkillers. A glass of wine, or six, won't do any harm, either.

...

I thought I was okay with the negative result from the AI — expecting it as I was — but really I'm not. Maybe I was more hopeful than I realised. I've only just started to accept that I can't fall pregnant naturally — now I'm wondering if I won't be able to fall pregnant with help, either.

I think the hardest thing for me is that all the right elements were there, but it still didn't work. I definitely ovulated, the sperm was good, the insemination was done at exactly the right time. Why didn't it bloody work? Is my uterus so deformed that it won't ever accept an embryo? Was there even an embryo, or is there something wrong with my eggs too? Surely the odds of my having bad eggs on top of everything else must be super slim? Or — I don't want to think this thought but it is hovering like a giant white balloon-animal elephant — maybe if some parts of my babymaker are faulty then other parts are likely to be faulty, too.

There are so many things that can go wrong, so many hurdles to stumble over, it's a wonder that anyone ever gets pregnant, whether they are the unfortunate owners of a slippy-slide or not.

IF vs. FI

I hesitate to call myself infertile and it's not because I'm in denial. I despise the word. It's so final, as if my body is broken beyond repair. When you hear that someone is infertile you don't picture them pregnant, do you? Or holding a baby? Well, I won't accept that. When I talk about my bum babymaker to friends I say, rather, that I have 'fertility issues' — in other words, I see it as a challenge to overcome and not a life sentence.

Semantics, a bit like differentiating between a victim and a survivor. Same scenario, different words, different energy. I believe in the power of words.

Not A Department Store

As a gesture to the universe (and, let's be frank, also to feel better about myself and assuage my debilitating broodiness) I've signed up as a volunteer at an orphanage in Westcliff. It's a well-run place with the cutest little bambinos. They're lovely to cuddle and it's balm to my soul. I get home smelling of baby powder and milk-vomit. Sometimes Mike comes with me. I love seeing him hold them. I wonder if this is the first step to adopting. There are at least a dozen I wouldn't think twice about taking home.

While volunteering you can't afford to bond too much because you never know if they'll still be there the next time you visit. You want them to be adopted, of course, that's the point, but there is a twinge of sadness when you realise a little pumpkin is missing. As soon as one leaves, his place is taken by a newborn. Some are prem and so very tiny; they need the most cuddling but are also the most vulnerable to volunteers' germs, so you need to be extra careful.

When I've done my bi-monthly four-hour Saturday shift I get home exhausted, smelly, and fulfilled. I feed enough babies and change enough nappies to get me through a week of living in an all-too-tidy baby-less home.

...

Mike hates the pain so much. He wishes there was something he could do to fix it. He sees my desolation. He watches the tears run down my face and wants to hit something.

HAPPY UN-BIRTHDAY

Not celebrating my birthday this year. Feel decidedly grinch-like. What is there to celebrate etc., etc.

Still upset that the AI didn't work. Wonder if anything will ever work. There are certainly no births in my immediate future. Happy un-birthday to me.

I am extremely bad at putting on a smiley-face when I feel sad, so best not to see too many people. Like a particularly responsible Ebola patient, I am selflessly deciding not to spread my flesh-eating misery. Will have a bottle of wine on my own instead. God, how sad, I hear you thinking. I agree. Cheers.

DING DONG!

I saw Micky today. She is happy with this journal. She doesn't read it — obviously — I just bring it along to show to her, like an overly-diligent schoolgirl with homework she doesn't want to admit she enjoyed doing. I think Micky was surprised by how much writing I'd done — she had perhaps been expecting a couple of one-liners. We can both see that it's helping me. At least I don't sit and cry for the full 60 minutes anymore.

She is, however, concerned that I don't have some kind of case manager. I have a psychologist and an acupuncturist and a reflexologist and a fertility specialist and a GP but no one is talking to anyone else and I'm the one left in charge. It would take some of the weight off my shoulders. I agree with her, but don't know how to resolve it. It's not like fertility case managers walk around knocking on your door like Jehovah's Witnesses.

SFX: DING DONG!

'Can we talk to you about Jesus Christ?'

'I don't know. Maybe. Can I talk to you about my broken babymaker?'

'Er … what now?'

'My babymaker. God gave me a broken one. I need an exchange. Or a refund. Or something. A baby will do, but make it a looker.'

'Er.'

'My husband and I have been having lots of sex — all kind of sex! — for over a year now and look, no swollen tummy. No milk jugs. No mewling newborn. What is up with that? Will you ask him? Jesus, I mean?'

(Awkward silence, in which I place my hands on my hips)

'I don't think ...'

'So you're saying Jesus can't help me, then?'

'It's not really our ...'

'So you're not going to become my case manager?'

'Your what-what?'

(The quiet, wide-eyed JW starts pulling the blushing JW away from the gate. A gust of wind blows his pamphlets out of his hand, littering the street with swirling God-confetti. They don't wave goodbye.)

19

HOLY FUCKING SHITBALLS

I learnt something today. I was chatting to Dani and she was telling me about the time that she had to go for an HSG — but she didn't get the memo to take painkillers beforehand. She said she was lying there, not suspecting a thing apart from some 'mild discomfort' when all of a sudden it felt like someone had reached into her uterus and was trying to turn it inside out.

She said she yelled out at the top of her voice: 'Holy Fucking Shitballs!'

When she told me the story, I couldn't help laughing. She said everyone in the room did the same thing.

In school, Pin had to have her wisdom teeth taken out. She was back almost immediately after the surgery, and even went to our house plays that night. When I had my wisdoms out a few years after that, I sat on the couch and cried the whole afternoon. I just sat there while tears streamed down my cheeks. Like a crying cry-baby. I know Pin is tough stock, with both English and Afrikaans (farmer) genes, but, really? Am I really such a wuss?

I want to be able to be flippant about pain, like they are. I want to be able to joke about it. And I want to stop taking all this shit so personally.

I learnt something today: I learnt to say Holy Fucking Shitballs.

My Infertility Doesn't Define Me

Wise and wonderful Roela came for tea. She was one of my favourite lecturers at college and I always love seeing her, but today my older sister from another mister was especially beneficent. We spoke about many things over home-made rusks, and then, of course, about my situation. Forever the soul of a teacher: she always has insightful words.

She told me that my infertility doesn't define me.

I knew that, but I think I needed to hear it from someone else.

I am a creative person and with my art, my garden, my writing, my life is the opposite of infertile. If I keep this in mind it keeps me from feeling like a dried-out husk. Despite my body's subtle betrayal, I am inherently fertile. She left some of her colour with me today.

It's such a simple idea. As soon as the words were

out of her mouth I was nodding. Yes, of course it doesn't, I know it doesn't, I said. But did I / do I? Why did it feel like she had reached out and taken something heavy off my chest? She said it a few times, to make sure I'd heard her, to make sure that the words had landed on my heart. Her eyes didn't let go of mine until she saw that I got it.

I got it. I got it, and feel lighter for it. It's a gift that will help me now and in the coming days. It also made me consider the concept of self-definition. What DOES define me? I am a book dealer, a listener, a reader, a baker, a gardener, a runner, a walker, a writer, a feminista, a daughter, an eater, a drinker, a sun-saluter, a lover, an enthusiastic list-maker. I am one-half of The Tag-Team of Love.

You are not defined by what you are not. A man does not define himself as a non-woman. So why say that I am non-fertile? Because, I sigh, it's there. It's important and it's undeniable. It may not define me, but it is my shimmering silhouette.

. . .

We were wondering if the pain medication is compromising my fertility. Mike suggested I try going one month without painkillers. I felt panicky, like I was about to have an anxiety attack, and then I started crying. Even with pills it is unbearable, I can't go without. I wish I could, if it would help our chances, but I know I can't.

Poor Mike. He married a strong, brave woman and is now saddled with a couch cry-baby. I've wept more this year than I have my whole life combined.

Mike: Hi Neets. How was your day?

Me: (FACE MELTS)

God, it makes me feel pathetic.

20

Don't Mention the War

We had dinner with Chris last night, up the road at Bottega. We were updating him on our treatment options and got around to discussing IVF. I told him how conflicted I feel about it, how I think it's wrong to spend so much on a (small) chance to conceive, how far that money would go in an orphanage, or to help support a poor family. He understood my dilemma, but didn't agree. He said that people are blowing similar amounts all the time on 'unnecessary' things like weekends away, designer handbags and ugly jewellery. Granted, these are rich and/or crazy people, but the point remains that our own money, spent mindfully by us on IVF, may grant me my ultimate wish, one that will last a lifetime.

I can't help but (conveniently) agree. If you want something badly enough, you can convince yourself of anything. What is money, anyway? A man-made construct to keep us all working and spending and in line. If I can't use the money I work so hard for (and as a bookseller and a writer, believe me, I work hard for my money) on the one thing in life I have always wanted, then what is the point (of anything)?

. . .

Dani has struggled with her fertility for years but finally fell pregnant a few months ago. I'm so happy and relieved for her. She knows I am in the thick of it and made me promise to read 'So Close' by Tertia Albertyn. I ordered it immediately.

She asked if I was seeing a fertility specialist, and I said yes. I told her that I think that I am in very good hands with the BFG and the fertility clinic he works in. She frowned. She knows a lot of clinics and doctors and didn't even know there was a fertility clinic at the hospital, and had never heard of the BFG. She said that I should go to her doc, who she absolutely loves, for a second opinion. I think her words were, 'He can make anyone pregnant. I wouldn't be surprised if he could make a man pregnant.'

I thought it would take a lot to get me to leave the BFG. He has been good to me and I feel loyal to him, but with a report like that of another specialist I was, like, 'See ya later!' I know how long Dani tried, how close she was to giving up, and now she is five months pregnant. The BFG can eat my dust.

. . .

Made an appointment to see Dr G at what seems to be SA's best fertility clinic. Have to wait for an appointment and it's going to be a very expensive second opinion.

So Close

Holy shit, this book. 'So Close' by Tertia Albertyn. Such heartache, such deep, bottomless sadness, and then triumph. Tertia is my superhero. An infertility warrior. After seven (7!) IVFs and losing a precious baby, she eventually gave birth to healthy twins. The book filled me with awe and fear. What if I am one of those cases that has to undergo so many IVFs? What if I lose a baby like Tertia did? I don't know if I can handle the pain. I could barely handle reading about it. Her steely resolve and barbed humour carries you along as she drags you by the scruff of your neck on her tumultuous journey.

I made Mike read it. It would be good, I thought, for him to really confront this thing. To know what's at stake. Towards the end of the book, when things start going wrong with her beautiful baby Ben, he started to sob. I was completely taken aback. In eight years I had never seen him cry.

The book has completely changed my mind about IVF. If that is my only option to conceive, then fuck it, I'll do it. If Tertia can do so many, and go through so much, then I can at least try it.

...

We saw Dr G today. I think I'm in love. I left thinking, if this man makes me pregnant, at least I can say that I loved the man who made me pregnant. He's like a cuddly bear.

The waiting room was absolutely crammed with a

mixture of hope and cynicism. You can see who the long-term patients are: the ones with the jaded looks on their faces. They don't glance at you as you walk in, they can't stand the newbies, with all their golden-sunshine-rays-of-hope emanating from their bodily orifices. If they had cigarettes they'd put them out on the newbies' foreheads, to remind them that life can suck, and suck badly, no matter how positive you are. So shut up.

When it's time to go in, we're ushered into an office to wait for the doc. Mike was hilarious. He looked at the fertility doll sculptures by the window and said 'I don't see any kind of accreditation on the walls. Do we know if this guy is even a doctor?' I almost wet myself I laughed so hard: behind him the entire wall was covered with framed certificates, degrees and awards. You could hardly see the wallpaper.

We both liked Dr G immediately. I told him our history and he dropped a few bombshells that completely changed our game plan.

1. Bicorniate Uteri are so rare that he could almost guarantee that it is not the case. His diagnosis after looking at the HSG (hysterosalpingogram) x-rays: a septate uterus. While the heart-shape is the same, the prognosis is (happily) vastly different. Bicorniates cannot be operated on with much success, but septums (the 'septum' is the actual cleft in the top of the heart, giving it its shape, dividing the uterus) are a piece of pie. You can cut those suckers out. This changes everything. I will no longer have a satanic womb.

2. Dr G thinks Mike's swimmers are A-okay. He

emphasised this, in my direction, as if I had been the one to imply that there was a problem in the first place. As if I had made up the whole Monster Sperm thing! Pssh! Anyway, this is awesome news.

3. My FSH (Follicle Stimulating Hormone) is sky-high, and my LH (Luteinising Hormone) is too low. This means that my eggs are running out. Not only are they in short supply, but if we're running on empty it probably also means that they are old and not very good quality. Ouch. He went as far as to say that I may have Premature Ovarian Ageing and we need to act fast. I seem to have haggard ovaries.

4. If I have endo on my diaphragm, then I almost certainly have it all over my babymaker. Endo is Very Bad News. This also changes everything. Fuck.

So, sitting there, we come up with a plan of action:

I'll need surgery. With my head spinning, we agreed to a date, despite it being the same month as the soccer World Cup.

Dr G tells us a little about endometriosis. It used to be called the 'career woman's disease' because it was usually diagnosed in older women. He said that most of the cases he sees are mainly due to couples deferring their baby-making till they're settled in career and home. It's the responsible thing to do in all ways but one: fertility-wise, it's foolish.

So I sit there with my withered ovaries and presumed endo, and think ... *I waited too long?*

Impossible.

Dr G says: 'so, basically, you waited too long.'

Gobsmacked. How is that possible, given my life-long broodiness and my sprinting towards conceiving as soon as I turned 30? I'm only 31 now. That's not ancient, is it?

Oh, the irony. My mother was worried that with me she'd have a teenage pregnancy on her hands, now she has an infertile daughter. Nice one, universe, I think, keep us guessing.

Our prognosis is in some ways better, and some ways worse, than we thought. But Dr G thinks he can make it happen. The overriding emotion is relief. If there is going to be someone who can get us pregnant, it's this doctor. We both trust him. I believe he will take care of us; after just one meeting I feel like this journey will be less lonely.

...

Dr G was so funny the way he went on about Mike's sperm yesterday. Because the BFG said that its morphology (shape) was 'problematic' (AKA Monster Sperm), I obviously brought it up in our first meeting. Dr G seemed horrified, as if I had, as they say, Mentioned The War. He said that the sperm was wonderful, the sperm was magnificent. Okay, I said, I've got it. The sperm could fertilise an entire African village, he insisted. Okay, Doc, settle down, I wanted to say. I am thrilled that you are so happy with the sperm. Don't feel that you need to wax lyrical about Mike's swimmers, please. His sense of masculinity does not rest entirely on the quality of his spermatazoa. He is more evolved than that. On the other hand, I am very excited that he has good sperm.

'It's better than 'good'!' The doc exclaimed, eyeing me with preacher eyeballs. Okay, Dr G, I (didn't) say: We get it. Now cut it out or get a room. You're making everyone feel uncomfortable.

...

The World Cup starts next month! Everyone now owns a vuvuzela. It sounds like South Africa has been invaded by giant mosquitoes with world-domination on their minds.

Our plan, with Mandie and Avish, is to watch as many live matches as possible. We bought as many tickets as we could, and for the other important matches we'll visit appropriate restaurants/bars and watch on TV.

Uruguay vs Mexico? We'll be chugging margaritas and eating nachos at that legit Mexican restaurant in Melville. Greece vs France: we have our eyes on Parea in Illovo. When we're at a loss for an ethnic place we'll go back to Melrose Arch where all the tourists hang out.

...

My brother's ex-girlfriend, D, phoned me to tell me she was pregnant with her new boyfriend's child. She was told a few years ago that she wouldn't be able to conceive so she didn't pay much attention to contraception and all of a sudden Whammo! She was knocked up. She is happy and I'm happy for her. She is lovely and deserves a lot of happiness. It still hurt, though.

21

A BLOWTORCH TO YOUR BABYMAKER

It's the World Cup! It's the World Cup! The country is going crazy with South African flags in any and every form. Rainbow wigs. Lighters. Car side-mirror socks.

We booked a long table at Central Station in the Melrose Arch square for the opening ceremony and first match and invited all our friends. We ordered beers the size of our arms and ate burgers and sang and danced.

...

My surgery — laparoscopy and hysteroscopy — is next week.

I have to sell my ticket for the Paraguay game — it's the day after the surgery.

I'm scared. I'm scared of being unconscious and cut open, scared of what they will find, and what could go wrong. At the same time, it feels good to take a drastic step to improve my fertility.

...

HOLY SHIT.

I was very nervous for the surgery, anxious of what they would find. Petrified that they would discover endo all over the place, or worse. This is kind of how my nightmares would go:

(Eyelids flicker open as the anaesthetic wears off. Three surgeons wearing blood-stained scrubs stand at my bedside. Shocked and exhausted, it looks like they've been wrestling with a particularly violent red-inked giant squid.)

'Mrs Lawrence, we opened you up, and what we discovered was, well, it was quite frightening, really.'

'What do you mean? Do I have endometriosis?'

'Pssh. We see endometriosis every day. Endo doesn't scare us. We laugh in the face of endo. We make silly faces and do interpretative dance when we see endo.'

(The three of them, despite being bone-weary, start making dopey faces, and dance. I shake my head to clear it, thinking it must be the pethidine in my IV that is making clowns of these doctors, but still they prance.)

'Okay, I get it. So ... there's a problem with my babymaker?'

'Mrs Lawrence, there is no easy way to say this. You don't even HAVE a babymaker. Where other women have babymakers, you have: - a) a cheap Chinese replica b) a jet engine c) a crossword puzzle or d) a toy T-rex dinosaur.'

'Well, which is it?'

'We couldn't really tell. But the point is, neither of those things can produce a sproglet.'

(They throw their clipboards over their shoulders.)

'But, surely, ...'

(They stick their fingers in their ears and sing 'La-la-la-la' until I stop talking.)

'Sorry we couldn't help. We're off to shower and then drink overpriced tequila. It's poker night.'

Luckily, the news was better than that - but not by much.

The morning started badly, when I discovered that my anaesthetist was a fuckhead. He interviewed me, used his stethoscope, and told me I had a heart murmur. I was already anxious for the surgery. Not one to overreact, I was, like, *what the FUCK?!* Then he had the nerve to look nervous. He listened again, and retracted his previous statement. So that is the story of how I was diagnosed with, then completely cured of, a heart murmur, in less than 30 seconds.

But that's not what made him a fuckhead. That came later. In the interview I told him I had an ulcer so he warned me that he would only be prescribing painkillers, no anti-inflammatories. He said it might be 'tough'. Last night I wanted to hunt the fucker down and burn his nether regions. It felt like my babymaker had been taken out, set alight, and put back again. My bladder was cramping. I didn't even know that was possible. I couldn't sleep. It's not that I battled to get to sleep, or that I slept badly: I didn't sleep at all, not for a minute. I ended up watching series on my laptop at 3am afraid that I would go insane if I didn't somehow distract myself.

I know I'm being emotional about him (the fuckhead/anaesthetist), but I really think he could have offered some kind of alternative to giving me only half the pain meds. There must be a hundred different anti-inflammatories out there that wouldn't have affected my ulcer.

Okay, back to the important stuff, like how the surgery went. I can tell I'm a bit loopy from lack of sleep by looking at what I've written so far. Ravings of a mad woman.

Mike dropped me off and I managed to get some work done, lying there in my hospital gown, seeing pale women get wheeled in and out of the operating room. I wondered what they were in for. Everyone seemed to have someone with them: husbands, sisters, mothers, best friends. I was the only one flying solo. That's if you don't count my laptop, which I sometimes do. I didn't mind. It made me feel stronger. I didn't need someone to hold my hand. I was a grown woman. Besides, Mike would be there when I woke up, I was sure.

Dr G was very sweet in the operating room. He told me he was going to fix me up and he held my hand while they knocked me out. When I woke up I wasn't in pain but felt cold and was shaking a lot. Mike wasn't there. I wasn't conscious enough to call a nurse and no one noticed so I lay there, shuddering, for what felt like ages, but was probably a few minutes. Soon my abs started waking up. I felt like I had done a thousand sit-ups. Then the pain started slowly seeping back into my body, and with that, wet warmth started flowing out. I was thinking, 'I'm haemorrhaging, I'm haemorrhaging, I'm bleeding out, but no one can see.' This, I realised, is why you have someone there to hold your hand.

Soon a nurse arrived and dispelled the drama with a cup of tea, a terrible margarine-cheddar sandwich, and a shot of pethidine. I could have kissed her on the lips for that pethidine. She checked under the blanket and if she was surprised by the amount of blood on the sheets, she didn't show it. She just cleaned me up like a baby, shoved about 10 new pads between my legs, and put a clean sheet on top. I wanted to take her and her beautiful meds home with me. I wanted to bless her and her kids and her kids' kids for generations and generations.

Mike arrived in time to see Dr G, who came to debrief us. He said the septum is history (yay!). The endo was far worse than he expected (with mild endo, laps usually take around 15 minutes, I was under for an hour and a half). It was everywhere, and it was advanced. 'Did you get it all?' I asked.

Yes, he nodded, he got it all.

WHO LEFT A CORPSE ON THE COUCH

Another sleepless night. Not as much pain, not nearly, but enough to keep me up. I haven't slept in more than 48 hours.

After the match, Mandie, Avish and Mike came home and we watched the surgery DVD together. It was like some kind of sci-fi war movie — the most intimate kind— these probes with mechanical hands moving in around veined membranes and shifting things around. Other probes cutting and burning away the diseased flesh. Smoke and slurping blood. We skipped the raspberry slushies, and the popcorn.

Looking at the state of my babymaker pre-lap: shadow-patterned with lesions, and adhesions sticking things together (the doc literally cut one of my twisted fallopian tubes free from its pink spiderweb) it really is no wonder that I haven't been able to fall pregnant. It was like it belonged on one of those warnings on an Australian cigarette pack: See exhibit A) Healthy lung (a perfect specimen, like glistening skinned salmon) and exhibit B) Cancerous lung (lump of coal). My poor sagging ovaries looked like they belonged to some 120-year-old moonshine-swilling, chain-smoking, heroin-chasing hermit. One was in particularly bad shape - so Mike calls it my 'smoker's ovary'.

I'm still really sore. I don't know what to do with myself so I lie on the couch and cry. Every now and then I take a break to make myself a cup of tea or curse the anaesthetist, but mostly I just lie here and cry. I'm sure I will sleep tonight; I'm completely exhausted. I'm still bleeding a lot — not sure where all this blood is coming from — surely a little snipped septum wouldn't bleed this much? Feeling drained in every way. Soon I'll be siphoned empty and Mike will come through to the lounge and be, like, 'Who left a corpse on the couch?'

It's not all bad, though. This pain is temporary. What is important is that THEY FIXED MY UTERUS! (Heart-shape is history! Huzzah!) and ablated the endo. Not only does that mean that I may now be able to fall pregnant, but NO MORE SHOULDER PAIN!

Can I say it again? NO MORE SHOULDER PAIN. NO MORE SHOULDER PAIN.

(When I am healed) I want to run naked in the streets and shout it out. No more dodgy ute, no slippy-slide, no more pain. My fertility-future lies before me like a shining road paved with little gold-foil chocolate blocks of sunshine.

I have a real chance of having a baby. I can't believe it's true. I am (not-so-tentatively) hopeful.

Due to the mixture of drugs and no sleep, I am also having vaguely entertaining hallucinations. Cocoa seems to have multiplied. There may be a rogue cat-cloner operating in the neighbourhood. Either that, or she is magic. She does look like she should belong to a witch. Or maybe there is just a glitch in the matrix — one that you can only see if you haven't slept in 3 days. She'll be lying in the garden, rolling in the sand as she likes to do, and then I'll walk to the kitchen and see her there, having a snack.

...

It has now been 72 hours without sleep. I have run out of series to watch and just stare into the darkness like a catatonic shell, hoping that if I lie still enough and try to switch off my brain, slow my breathing, that it will be like sleep. I've tried to read but the words swim and I end up reading the same page over and over again. I didn't know it was possible to be awake for so long. It's not the pain keeping me awake, because even when it is under control I can't sleep. It's the strangest thing. Sleep has always come easily to me.

And the bleeding. The bleeding and the bleeding. Where does all this blood come from? How am I not dead? My body has turned into this magic factory that runs on no blood and no sleep. The sunlight hurts my eyes. Perhaps I have turned into a vampire. Perhaps the next time I look in a mirror my reflection will no longer be looking back at me. Or maybe the reason the reflection has disappeared is because I really am dead. Died from that haemorrhaging in the hospital bed when no one could hear me shivering. That's why Mike talks less to me now, because I'm a ghost, and you can only talk so much to a ghost.

22

Up Beaver Creek

Today was a Holy Fucking Shitball of Shitballs day. Since having the surgery, I have had more shoulder pain.

The same amount of shoulder pain I had before the surgery.

What. The. Actual. Fuck.

When it started, I thought I was imagining it. I saw the DVD for God's sake! They lasered the fuck out of my insides. But there it was, in all it's Holy Fucking Shitball glory. But then what the BFG said came back to me — that you can't get all the diaphragmatic endo via a laparoscopy. And you can't lift the liver with those sci-fi probey things they use for a lap. So that's why he recommended abdominal surgery which I abhorred the idea of and conveniently forgot as soon as Dr G held my hand and told me he'd fix me.

I think I started seeing Dr G as my golden ticket out of this foggy nightmare. My knight in shining armour. Everything he said seemed right, proving the BFG wrong. But on a deeper level I think I knew it was too good to be true. How could one surgery fix the host of problems I have? If you have a misshapen uterus and endo all over your insides ... is it really possible to go into an operating room and come out 90 minutes later with babymaker just-serviced and purring? I think I knew the answer was no, but was so desperate to believe otherwise that I didn't think twice about chugging the Kool-Aid.

But all is not lost, I told myself, through those (psychologically) difficult days of pain. At least the heart-shape is fixed and the pelvic endo is gone. In theory, I should now be able to conceive. And if I can conceive, the pain will stay away. The diaphragmatic endo is still there, but we can deal with it later — once I have had my baby — if it is still a problem.

So, we have a follow-up with Dr G. He is happy that the surgery went really well. I told him I still had shoulder pain, and asked if he was able to treat my whole diaphragm (under my liver), and he said no, which I knew. He looked a little nonplussed at the question. He showed us a highlights package of the surgery DVD, explaining the important parts, like how he zapped that septum and freed up that tangled tube and ovary.

Most importantly, we spoke about our plan of action. It's relatively common for women with mild to moderate endo to fall pregnant in the months following a lap, so that is what we are hoping for, despite my endo being neither mild nor moderate.

We'll do medicated cycles, which means hormone pills, to force me to ovulate. Once I reach a certain day in my cycle they'll scan me to make sure that I am ready to ovulate, and then I'll be given a trigger shot (same as in AI/IUI) to make sure it happens within a certain window. Because there is no problem with Mike's swimmers, we'll try the old Have-Actual-Sex to get pregnant. I obviously find this a great deal more appealing than the turkey baster method. The doc calls the sex method 'doing your homework'. Guess I'll start calling Mike 'my homework'.

We will try for a couple of cycles, but only a couple, because endo is a vicious boomerang of a disease and will be back in no time. To add to that deadline, Dr G said my latest blood tests had shown that my egg quantity (and therefore, usually, quality) is on the decline, so we need to act fast. We didn't talk about what would happen if the medicated cycles don't work. Cross that bridge etc. etc., but I can't not think about it. I have to have some kind of plan to feel that I have some small measure of control over this thing.

I think that is one of the reasons I am finding infertility so difficult. In the past, if I worked hard at something and dedicated myself to it, I usually did quite well. No matter how hard I try to have a baby, it's just not happening. It's no surprise that it's people like me, Type A, who get endo. It's like the universe is saying to us: 'You may think you do, but you don't actually control ANYTHING.'

Just to prove the universe's point, we go down to have a follow-up HSG to look at my beautifully boring new regular-shaped uterus. I lie on the table, ready to 'Ooh!' and

'Aah!' at the screen. I didn't know about the HSG so I didn't take painkillers in time. I popped one as soon as I knew — a few minutes before — and hoped it would kick in quicksmart. At least there are some advantages, I thought, of carrying around schedule 5 painkillers in your handbag.

Mike was holding my hand when they injected the dye. At first I didn't understand what was happening — why were they showing old pictures on screen? I was sure that it was my 'before' shot. Were they doing it to compare? No, this was in real time. The dye was showing a very familiar, very distinct heart-shape, as if it hadn't had a makeover at all. And while my brain was scrambling, I got the mother of all cramps. It was like someone was using my uterus as a stress-ball. I instinctively put my hands over my stomach, obscuring the picture on screen. I saw the solid metal of my rings. They asked me to move my hands away. I whispered 'Sorry. Sorry,' and took them away. Stared blankly at the hateful heart on the screen. Wanted to punch it. Felt like someone *was* punching it. And then, when I remembered: 'Holy Fucking Shitballs,' but no one heard me.

. . .

Although I am not usually one for tantrums, I did come close to throwing one once I got off that HSG table. I was so furious I couldn't talk. I was shaking and trying to not cry. Mike tried to comfort me and I dissolved into a veritable salt-water Vesuvius.

How could it be? How could it be that after that traumatic surgery, I am still in as much pain as ever, and my uterus is still wonky? Standing there, confused, upset, dye running out of me, I wanted to shake my fist at the doctors and nurses and demand answers.

Dr G wasn't there for the HSG, so another doctor answered our questions. Yes, this was unfortunate, he agreed, but it's just a small step backwards, and won't change my overall prognosis. It's an inconvenience, but the big picture remains the same. AN INCONVENIENCE? I wanted to shout. I ALMOST DIED! (which was a bit melodramatic, even for me). Okay, fine, I'll knock it down a notch to I FELT LIKE I WAS DYING, which really isn't the same thing at all.

No, this doesn't happen often, said the doc, speaking calmly over my shouty thoughts: a septum that grows back after being excised is so rare that they don't even discuss the possibility with patients. Oh well then! Lucky me!

So I need another surgery — this time just a hysteroscopy — which requires no external cutting (they just go up beaver creek). Another general anaesthetic, another hospital bill that medical aid won't touch, another day or two off work, another week of bleeding.

After the HSG I had a meeting at an ad agency. Since Pulp has been doing well I haven't done much freelance copywriting — I haven't had the time nor inclination — but a friend there needed a copywriter on an urgent job and now I need the extra cash. Also, it is a great brand to work on (think of a certain popular Portuguese peri-peri chicken) and the job looked like it would be fun.

I was sitting in the boardroom, getting briefed, trying to concentrate, hoping that any evidence of the earlier tantrum was washed off my face, when I got more cramps and felt the rest of the dye streaming out of my nethers.

I sat as still as I could, hoping that the giantess-sized pad they had given me at the clinic would absorb most of it. I thanked whatever fashion god made me decide on dark jeans that morning, and whatever interior designer god made the agency choose plastic chairs for their boardroom. After the briefing I waited for as many people as possible to leave the room without arousing suspicion — asked if I could quickly check my email before leaving — and then when (I hoped) no one was watching, walked very carefully out of the building.

It seems then that my 'fertility issues' are bullshit and I am, indeed, infertile.

First Email Attempt Ever

Today my dad sent his first email, ever. It was to me.

Here it is, verbatim:

Hi Neets,

Missed you at the Radium on Sunday. How's the studying going? We think of you every day and more than hope that things work out the way you and Mike want them to. There are lots of us out here who love you very much and want the best possible result. As the Poms said in WWTwo, "Keep your chin up chaps."

With all my love,

Dad.

DEEP, DARK HOLE

I realised that I have been feeling incredibly resentful towards the fertility doctors, and fertility treatments. Because I (intensely) resent my infertility, I have been unfairly passing that negative emotion on to the only people who can actually help me.

I resent having to get help to do something that I should be able to do easily.

I resent having to pay them so much money for what should be a basic human right.

I resent the unnatural process of assisted reproduction.

I resent that procedures don't always work as they should.

But where would I be without fertility doctors? At the bottom of a deep, dark hole.

...

This time the surgery was a cinch. After all my tantrum-throwing about having to go in again, it was lovely to be able to go under and take a lovely long nap (haven't been sleeping well — knife in shoulder). Because there was no cutting into abdominal muscle there was hardly any pain — at most a few mild cramps, like a normal period — and because it is impossible to say no to pethidine when it is offered to you (especially after a few days of walking around with said knife in shoulder), I floated out of there feeling that all was right with the world. Ah, opiates, the world would indeed be a sad place without them.

23

MIKE JNR

We call our unborn (or, more correctly, un-conceived) baby 'Mike Jnr'. It's shorthand for our (nowadays brittle) dream of having a baby. It helps to have a name. It makes him seem more real, less of a fantasy. It also helps in writing email updates to friends and family — keeps it light. Subject: 'Update on Mike Jnr!' instead of: 'Feeling poor, sad and hopeless. Send schedule 16 painkillers.'

I've always written my goals in the sand. Before I started my business, when I was 'stuck' in advertising, I used to write 'Pulp' in the wet sea sand. Before that it was 'Mike'. Now I write 'Mike Jnr' at every opportunity I get. It's my way of committing it to the universe, making the wish more tangible. Mike calls it 'collapsing the possibility'.

It's been 18 months of writing it in the sand, and now I am less particular about where I scribble his name: steamed up mirrors, books, chalkboards, paper notes that get buried in the garden. I commit it over and over again to the earth. It may seem silly, but I feel that it has a certain power.

24

THE FERTILITY CAVE

Mandie and Avish weren't sure what to get me for my birthday. They knew all I wanted was a baby so they got creative. (No, they didn't kidnap a newborn, although they assure me that they did consider it.)

Instead they organised and sponsored a weekend away in Clarens for Mike and I. A weekend dedicated to conceiving. Not (necessarily) a dirty weekend, but to visit the fertility cave there. How they even knew about the cave, I can't guess. Mandie is on every contraceptive known to man and mammal. She was conceived while her mother was on the pill, so she takes no chances. While she is really good with babies, if you ask her if she wants one she slaps you with a glare that would freeze lava.

So last night we packed our bags and headed out to the Free State. I would never say no to a weekend away, and Clarens is so beautiful with its golden mountains, but I don't hold much hope for a miracle from some dirty cave that (I'm guessing) someone once thought looked like a giant vagina.

But we have gone from 'Not Trying' to 'Trying Absolutely Everything' and if that includes a punani grotto, then I'm in. My only objective this weekend is to have fun, and an open mind.

...

The pilgrimage didn't start well. It's not that the cave isn't well signposted, it's not signposted AT ALL. We drove around with no clue where we were going and I couldn't help feel that it was a cruel and apt metaphor for our fertility journey so far.

At first I couldn't bear to ask someone. I was sure no one would know, anyway. But we were about to give up and I couldn't go back to Jo'burg without having visited the cave. The first few people regarded us with confusion, and vague suspicion, (*Fertili-what-what?*) But eventually someone knew what we were talking about and pointed us in the right direction.

We finally found a little sand road that we had missed the first 23 times we had driven past. We picked up some pedestrians who we bribed to show us the way. I was worried they may be axe-murderers, leading us to a dead-end in order to rob us of our meagre possessions. The trip included going through a gate that warned you to not enter. We were, like, 'Are you sure this right?' and the guys were like 'Yes!' and we were, like, 'We are so going to get axed.'

We pulled into a makeshift parking lot in the middle of a huge herd of sheep. Two or three cars, but not a cave or another person in sight. We watched the sheep for a while, not sure what to do, when we saw people walk past us and making their way up the hill. That's when we realised that we would be working hard for our little bit of fertility magic: we had to hike to get to the cave.

I don't know what I was expecting. Perhaps something like the virility cave we saw in Thailand: a short, easy walk on a beach and *voila!* a huge cave full of phallic symbols. You giggle and admire them while someone chops open a coconut cocktail for you.

The hike was long and steep, and we weren't dressed for it, so we were hot and a bit grumpy on our way up. I was surprised at how many people were also walking the path. They were dressed in church gear and carried staffs, so we guessed the caves held more enchantment than just of the fertility variety.

Eventually we reached the top and hopscotched over a river to get to the cave, and it was as though we had crossed into another world. It wasn't as much a cave as it was a hobbit warren. Built into the recesses were tiny little interconnected dwellings with tiny little hobbit-sized doors (I kept my eyes peeled for hobbits, but no such luck). Instead, there were ordinary-looking humans walking around, among goats, dogs, cats and chickens. The closest thing I could find to a hobbit was a sweet little boy, around 3 years old, with an easy smile and dusty feet. He followed us, pointing things out. He let me pick him up and carry him while we explored. His parents didn't seem to be around, and I briefly considered taking him home with us, day-dreamed about looking after him. Then I remembered that kidnapping was illegal and I imagine that if getting pregnant outside of jail was this tricky, the chances of it happening while locked up might be even trickier. It would take a lot of planning to get Mike to pay a conjugal visit at exactly the right time of the month.

'Warden, please, I have to see my husband right now. Like, right now. In the next hour at the latest.'

(I facepalm myself for not thinking ahead and ordering KFC for her lunch today).

'Er, no. Get back to pulling out those blackjacks.'

'You don't understand. It's my window. (Whispers:) My ovulation window.'

(Warden slaps some sense into me.)

'Blackjacks!'

The hobbit houses were immaculate, and swept to within an inch of their lives. This wasn't some kind of (inconvenient) place to squat, it was clearly revered as some kind of holy place. There was a shrine, oily with years of molten wax, where we said a quick Hail-Mary or some-such. I've never been good with religion or bowing to man-made edifices, but I was wearing my Open Mind. After looking around in fascination and petting the odd smelly goat, we were shown to the Fertility Lady's place. She made us wait outside while she did what I guessed was some preparatory voodoo.

When she was ready for us, she called us in. We're not the shortest couple: we had to make ourselves hobbit-sized by folding ourselves in half and walking in on our knees. It was clearly a place of miracles: the fact that we all fitted in such a tiny space was a special kind of sorcery.

The interior was dim, cramped, and completely pimped. An array of fertility icons gleamed in the candlelight. The lady started off by chanting and dusting me (with what I guess was a feather duster with special powers and not a regular one from the local Shoprite/Checkers) and singing a bit. Then she put her hands on my stomach and pressed quite hard. Mike and I couldn't look at each other, afraid to offend her by laughing. She picked up a picture of a (white) mother nursing a baby, in a silver frame. I wondered if only white people came to ask her for help. She cradled the frame like an infant, rocking it, and kissed it, then passed it to me to do the same, making kissy noises. I cradled it, and it made me feel like I was a child again, playing in an (especially eccentric) friend's dollhouse.

Next came the really fun part: She produced an old, scratched plastic bottle (Sprite? Stoney?) filled with dirty water. Mike looked worried, but I wasn't nervous. I thought she might sprinkle it around us like holy water. Holy Fertility Cave Water. But it turned out that Mike had good reason to be twitchy. She poured some out into an enamel mug and passed it to me, motioning for me to drink it. I thanked her and pretended to take a sip, making sure my lips weren't anywhere near the filthy stuff, but she had clearly seen this trick before and got really bossy about me drinking it all. I looked for somewhere I could tip it out but the place was so tiny and she was staring right at me so there was no way I wouldn't be busted. At her insistence, I took a sip (I know! Hepatitis C. Cholera. There would be no getting pregnant now. But what choice did I have?). It was ice cold and tasted of sand and candle wax. I shudder to think of where it came from and was sure that I'd be rolling around in agony with some kind of vicious stomach bug that night. I was suddenly sure that this woman wanted me to puke all my evil infertile guts out. And I had fallen for it! Dammit!

Fortunately (for me) she then turned her attention to Mike. She took some of the freezing water and, wait for it, POURED IT INTO HIS EAR. He wasn't expecting it (obviously), and certainly wasn't expecting it to be so damn cold, and he screamed. A proper scream that reverberated on the close clay walls. Oh my God, I laughed so much I almost wet my shorts. I laughed and laughed. I was almost hysterical. Trying to not laugh made me laugh more. He tried to shake the water out of his eustachian tube (this is where his surfing experience should have come in handy) but the magic (read: filthy) water was there to stay. After all the commotion she still wanted to pour water in his other ear. And he let her. And he screamed again. I was finished.

Then it was my turn again, giving Mike a moment to shake and smack his head like someone deranged. She gave me the whole bottle of water, told me to drink it all (thankfully not right there and then, but rather as homework) and then put a shiny plastic tiara on my head. I will never forget that picture in my mind of Mike trying to get the water out of his ears and me, in a tiara, cuddling and kissing a picture of some stranger's baby, trying to stifle my maniacal laughing. If it had happened anywhere else I'm sure we would have been given straitjackets and our own padded cells.

At last we were let out into the sunshine, and we scrabbled in our pockets for cash. We weren't expecting an actual person or ritual, just an old cave, so we didn't bring our wallets on the hike. We only had a couple of notes and coins (certainly not enough for a miracle, we were sure) and handed them over sheepishly. I think she had expected more, explaining that the money was for 'the angels', but we didn't have anything else to give.

The little boy had waited outside for us and was happy to see us again, but when he realised we were going home he started crying. We both gave him a hug and told him not to cry, which made him cry more.

We said goodbye and ran down the hill, our spirits high from all the strangeness and laughing. We passed a *bliksem*-drunk man on his way up, tried to give him a wide berth, but that didn't stop him from shouting some slurry profanities in our direction. Nothing like a dirty drunk to bring you back down to earth.

In the car Mike was, like, 'I can't believe you drank that siff water.'

I was, like, 'Me neither!'

'That was not a good idea.'

'I think I've got Hepatitis.'

'You'll be lucky if that's all you've got,' he said, and I agreed, and we laughed some more as we tried to not run over any sheep on our way out.

BABY BEN!

To our great surprise the water didn't make me ill (that I know of, although I can picture little seahorse-shaped barbed-amoeba creatures attached to the inside of my intestines, having a good chomp at whatever comes their way) and we had a lovely night out at dinner.

We I woke up to a message on my phone, saying that Pin's baby had arrived. What wonderful, wonderful news. It's as if the fertility magic did happen after all, just not for me.

We drove back to Jo'burg and stopped for a quick shop on our way home. My phone buzzed and it was a picture of baby Ben. He looked so very perfect, so absolutely PERFECT, with his little button nose, and I thought he looked so much like my dear friend who I missed so much, that my face started leaking all over the place. Right there, in the homeware section of Woolworths, in-between slotted spoons and ornamental buddhas and tea towels, I gazed at my phone and did my Ugly Cry.

No Crying Over Bad Eggs

I had some more blood tests done. I thought that even though the rest of my fertility was trash, I hadn't yet heard anything TOO bad about my eggs, and happily (naïvely) assumed that they were A-okay. Or at least okay enough to be able to conceive. Dr G had other ideas.

'Look, guys, there is no delicate way to say this.'

'Spit it out, doc, we can handle it. Probably heard worse.'

'You're old.'

'We're not old! We're thirty-one! That's like the new twenty! We're still shiny!'

'You're old on the inside. Not shiny on the inside. Old and shrivelled.'

'That's a bit harsh.'

'Have you *seen* the state of your babymaker? I have. And it's Not Pretty.'

'Wow, feel free to not sugarcoat the truth.'

'We don't have time for sugar. We don't know how long you have before your endo comes back. Plus, your eggs are running out. They're not great eggs by any stretch of the imagination, but at least while you've still got some, we've still got something to work with.'

My baby cannon cringes. She's had enough of the barrage of insults. No wonder she is feeling hollow-cheeked.

So my eggs, apart from being rare, are past their sell-by date. Not a good combination. It's not the end of the world, it just means that whatever we plan to do, we need to do it as quickly as possible. There is no time to cry over bad eggs. There's been plenty of crying over dodgy uteri and tangled up nether-organs: no more tears now. It's time for action. Every month that passes literally lowers our chances. He recommends three timed cycles starting now (a month after the surgery). I've a had a bit of a springclean down there and a septum snip so there's a chance they'll work. If they don't, we'll go straight to IVF.

Without even discussing it between ourselves, Mike and I both nodded decisively at the doc. All the conversations we have had about reasons to not do IVF vanished from our collective memories. Yes, we nodded, let's get on with this thing.

'Okay,' we agreed, 'we don't want to wait too long.'

Dr G looked at us. 'You're here because you already waited too long.'

25

BAD PIÑATA

Despite the bad news about my eggs, and the inevitability of a (previously dreaded) IVF in our future, our spirits are buoyed. I'm going to get rid of this pain. I'm going to get pregnant. How good it feels to have a plan. We're ready. Let's do it. Let's punch it in the face. Let's hit it like a bad piñata.

26

My Therapist Broke Up With Me

Today my therapist broke up with me. She said that we have discussed everything at length, and that I seem to be handling, so she doesn't want to waste my time or money with further sessions until I feel that I need one (i.e. she is bored to death of my infertility and would rather see her more interesting clients, the ones with multiple personalities and kinky sex hang-ups). She said to keep on with this journal and see her when I feel the need to. On one hand I agree with her, on the other I feel that I may need her more than ever if we have to go through with IVF. It made me feel good though, strong.

Commitment is Scary

We went to Sue and Stu's engagement party today. Theme: Halloween, because Commitment Is Scary! There we are, all milling around in their sunny garden, vampires and gremlins and pregnant schoolgirls, clutching our cold beers and eating crisps, when Stu's sister stands up to thank us for coming, and lets us know that the engagement party is now over. We were all, like, Cookie Monster 'huh?' and then she said 'Because it's now their WEDDING!' and then the music starts and Sue is walking down the 'aisle' of Frankensteins and long-haired witches and there is a Pagan lady with a robe and next thing they have jumped the broom and tied the knot. Stu hugged his corpse bride so hard it brought tears to my eyes.

Shortest engagement everrr. Everyone was so hopped up by the surprise and the emotion that it turned out to be one of the best parties. At home, I stripped off my skeleton stockings and removed my Clockwork Orange eyelash while my mind was still boggling.

...

Finally we get to do a timed (medicated) cycle, after that small hiccup of a month's delay due to the miraculously resilient/stubborn septum. This time we did an out-patient hysteroscopy in the doc's office (just a camera) and we all sighed in relief when we saw that the septum was really, truly, gone.

If all is okay with the scan on day 3 I'll start popping the meds and we'll start our 'homework' when we get the go-ahead from Dr G. It's time to make this happen!

TMI

I know this is a journal, and shouldn't really require a Too Much Information warning, but I am thinking of my future self reading this page. Maybe I won't want to be reminded of the more 'candid' aspects of fertility treatments. Maybe I won't want to re-live the gory bits. Or maybe someone else has the cheek to read my private entries, in which case they deserve to be warned, despite their transgression.

Either way, you have been alerted. Just skip this part. Turn the page now. Like internet porn, you have to be cautious: once you see something dodgy you cannot, ever, un-see it.

I went in for my Day 3 scan today (Day 1 is the first day of your period), to make sure that all is quiet down there so that we can start the medicated cycle. They check that nothing is inflamed, there are no cysts, etc. So although I am no longer a stranger to the dildo-cam, the nurse shows me into the room and tells me to take off my panties: I was, like, Oh shit! I can't have a dildo-scan! I've got my period! But the nurse just laughed and said that was normal for a Day 3 scan. I was aghast. They wanted me to take out my tampon and lie (and maybe bleed) on their table? They were going to use the dildo-cam even though it would come out bloody?

Eeewwyuck. I really didn't want to. I know there are those women who celebrate menstruation: they don't baulk at period-sex, they have first-period-parties replete with uterus-shaped piñatas, vajayjay cupcakes and games of pin-the-ovary-on-the-fallopian tube, they paint feminist slogans on canvasses in their menstrual blood, they knit scarves from stained wool spooling from — ahem — You Know Where. I'm not one of them. The idea that someone I'm not even intimate with is going to see my blood makes me cringe. I don't even look at my own blood. I'm sure you could psychoanalyse the hell out of this. I'm sure you could say that no wonder I have endo if my feminine energy is so blocked that I can't face my own period.

You could also try to reason with me, saying that these doctors have seen my baby cannon inside and out (well, that made me cringe too), that they have seen THE INSIDE OF MY UTERUS, so what is the problem with a bit of blood?

Thank God those scan rooms are dimly lit. I just looked away when it was over and pretended nothing was out of the ordinary. I may have whistled a little tune. It was mortifying. What about the nurses who had to clean me like a baby after the surgeries? That was also mortifying. Shouldn't I be used to these small humiliations by now? Yes, but I'm not. You wait, I hear people say in my head, Just You Wait until you Give Birth. Yes, well, stupid people in my head, I'd love to.

Anyway (brushing that under the carpet!) we got the green light for our first timed, medicated cycle and I am now on Femara. It can supposedly have all kinds of dodgy side effects, like back pain, bone pain, muscle pain, hot flushes, anxiety, etc., etc., but I feel okay. My shoulder was sore for a bit longer than usual, which is understandable, seeing as it is aggravated by hormones and I'm taking extra. But it wasn't too bad and all in all it hasn't been difficult.

I'm feeling better about everything, actually. I've had the surgeries, I'm all cleaned up Down There, I'm definitely going to ovulate, and I have an amazingly good-looking sperm donor on hand. This might be the month I fall pregnant. I know, I know, it's a long shot, but there is a chance. Every day this month is brightened by that glimmer.

Have you ever seen the Starbucks espresso ads? They won at Cannes a while back. I cannot watch them without laughing. Something about the over-the-top humour appeals so much to me.

I love the 'Glen' (Eye of the Tiger) execution, but my favourite is the one in the open-plan office where everyone is completely hopped up on caffeine. Hilarious! My copywriter at Jupiter used to joke that I was like the broody female character (crazy-eyed: "Babies Everywhere!" she shouts, while stuffing her cardigan full of office supplies, to look pregnant.) He used to act it out in our office and we'd piss ourselves. I loved working with him, he'd always make me laugh. He did especially good impersonations of Doctor Evil from Austin Powers. We did some good work together and were very close. "Babies Everywhere!"

All of which reminds me of one of his (many) pearls of infinite wisdom, which has stood me in good stead:

"If you don't laugh, you cry." — Stephen Anderson

27

THE HOSTILES, OR, ANGRY VAGINAS

The humiliation continues. Part of this first medicated cycle is to have a PCT: Post-coital test. This does not involve, as you may think, a pub-like pop quiz after a good shag. Instead, we are to 'do our homework' during our ovulation window, and go to the clinic first thing the next morning (without showering) to witness how Mike's swimmers are faring up the creek.

Apparently there is such a thing as 'hostile cervical mucous'. It means that the cervical environment is acidic and, as you can guess, not good for sperm.

A test! I feel completely unprepared. Should I be eating more yoghurt, or something?

PCT = EPIC FAIL

I'm going to go out tonight to drink a vast amount

of whisky. Okay, I'm in the middle of a medicated cycle so I'll just have one and make my friends do the rest of the drinking for me. As you have probably gathered, the PCT did not go well. In fact, it couldn't have gone any worse.

So we're there in the room at the clinic, blinking weary eyes, so early that neither of us have even registered that it's morning. The doc takes a swab and smears it on the little glass slide and puts it under the microscope, which shows us what is happening on the big screen adjacent to it. That woke me up.

I think my jaw hung open for a while, as Dr G sort of gathered himself and started talking. I didn't hear anything for those first few minutes. My attention was completely focused on the massacre before my eyes: all I could see were hundreds of dead or dying sperm. The dead soldiers were one thing — ghost-sperm! — but watching the others writhe and struggle and swim in wounded circles was just too much. And I was the one who had maimed and killed them. I could almost hear them groaning in agony. In my imagination one particularly brave tadpole, shivering in the beginning of his death throes, urges the rest of his squad to go on without him.

I've said it before, I'll say it again. What. The. Fuck.

I had given the poor things an acid bath — they never stood a chance.

'Never' being the operative word that makes this difficult to accept: Of all the months of 'not trying,' followed by the months of 'really trying': taking my temperature, prodding my body for signals, the carefully-timed ovulation-window sex ... of all those months (18 failed cycles), all that hope that was dashed, over and over again, and all that pain, and actually, there had never been a chance. THERE HAD NEVER BEEN A CHANCE.

I feel like I've been swiped sideways. I feel like (emotionally-speaking) I was walking down the street, perfectly alive, and some asshole in a BMW skipped a stop sign and sent me flying. Irrationally, I felt the need to apologise to Mike. I thought that if someone had killed thousands upon thousands of *my* soldiers I would at least expect a card and a fruit basket.

'Wow,' I said, when I finally regained my ability to speak. 'That's not good.'

I expected Dr G to don a hazmat suit and usher me out of his building. It was clear that I was radioactive and a hazard to the general population.

I expected him to say: 'Holy Moses! I've never seen such a gruesome slaughter. Who would have guessed that a seemingly benevolent vagina could be responsible for such annihilation?' and then: 'Would you mind if we took you and your cervical environment along to our next PCT WTAF conference? I'm sure the fraternity will find your mucous entirely fascinating.'

Instead he recommended I douche with bicarb. I was, like, do what with what-what? I have never douched in my life. I thought douching had gone the way of trepanning and toothbrush moustaches. I thought the last people to douche were promiscuous French women in the 1800s. I thought only people with a severe form of OCD would even consider douching nowadays; it's an old wives tale that I have absolutely no interest in trying. He said the alkalinity of the bicarb should neutralise the acidity of the CM, creating a less hazardous playground for the swimmers. Those poor guys. I don't want to be the fertility version of Idi Amin. It looks like I have no choice but to try it.

TMI: Project Douche

Tools required:

1x (larger-than-expected) douching instrument (syringe with bulb) (Strange-looking thing - I think I may have gasped when the nurse whipped it out of her supplies cupboard. I was, like, Holy Moly! What the hell is that thing?)

1x warm bath

1x box of bicarbonate of soda (or, in Afrikaans, Koeksoda! Koek, get it? Hee.)

1x teaspoon

1x glass beer tankard that you will never drink out of again. Not because it goes anywhere near your — ahem — hostile mucous, but because every time you see it you will be reminded of the not-romantic exercise of irrigating your punani.

Also handy: supreme gymnastic talent, or, lacking that, a developed sense of humour.

Method:

1. Run a shallow bath. Not too hot. Hot baths are bad for fertility. Jesus Christ, don't you know anything?!

2. Mix one heaped teaspoon of bicarb with one tankard of warm water. Don't be distracted by the logo on the tankard. This is not the time to think about having a nice cold beer.

3. Get in bath.

4. Use the bulb syringe to suck up bicarb solution from the tankard.

5. Kind of angle yourself backwards, on your haunches, while simultaneously holding on for dear life and squirting the solution up your nethers. This requires a reasonable amount of dexterity and determination.

6. Relax, and let it out.

7. Repeat steps 5 and 6 as many times as you need to, to finish the solution, trying to not pull any muscles or slip and brain yourself on porcelain.

8. While practising your unique form of douche-yoga, accidentally knock over the box of bicarb so that it lands in a puddle of spilt bathwater. Swear a little. Crave a cigarette, even though you haven't smoked in five years.

9. Try again. In the middle of a particularly challenging pose, you hear footsteps outside the bathroom. As if caught in a lewd act, you immediately drop everything and start whistling.

10. When your husband comes in, you sit on the bulb syringe to hide it, and pretend to drink the bicarb solution out of the tankard.

11. 'Staying hydrated!' you shout at him, in case he doesn't buy it. You add an enthusiastic thumbs-up and smile with all your teeth.

12. He looks at you as if you are insane. There is a little fear in his eyes. He backs out the bathroom door, perhaps even the front door, grabbing his toothbrush and sleep shorts on his way.

13. When it is over, lie back in the cold, quimmy water and wonder what the hell your life has come to. A pre-sexy-time bath used to consist of a glass of red wine, baby oil, and scented candles. Stare at the brightly-lit bulb syringe and feel suitably depressed.

14. Now snap out of it! Time to feel sexy! Forget that you just used a common baking ingredient to neutralise your acid bath of a vagina, and hope that your husband decided to stick around.

15. Hubba-hubba, bow-chick-a-wow-wow, etc.

HIGH-FIVING MY CERVIX

Another PCT today. (Waking up when it's still dark to sit in traffic to come to a clinic to wait in a waiting room to have your pootang swabbed and then put under a microscope is so awesome.)

This time we passed. I watched the screen through my fingers, not being able to take another battleground scene — I sense that the first one will forever haunt me, to the soundtrack of 'Saving Private Ryan' — but yay for old wives tales and bulb syringes: the swimmers were alive! I felt like high-fiving my cervix.

The Hostiles, or, Angry Vaginas

Mike has taken to calling my CM 'The Hostiles' (from the TV series 'Lost').

So now, douching has become 'taking out The Hostiles'. Sometimes, during sex, I picture a tribe of creepy island survivors camping out on the dirty upside-down hill of my cervix. It's them against The Swimmers.

My female friends and I refer to hostile cervical mucous as 'Angry Vagina'. The first time I heard the phrase I spat sangria out of my nose.

'I also have an Angry Vagina!' says an acquaintance at a party, chinking my glass of wine. Forget the First Wives Club, we're the Angry Vaginas. And there are a lot of us. Does naturally sperm-friendly CM even exist? we wonder out loud to each other in someone's kitchen at a party. If it does, I bet it's as rare and difficult to harness as a unicorn's fart.

I referred to my Angry Vagina the other day in company not yet familiar with the term, and she spilled her drink out of her nose, too.

Nose-irrigation: the initiation ceremony for Angry Vaginas all over the world.

28

CHURNING OF THE SEA

Mandie, Avish, Mike and I decided to have an impromptu break in Slaap-Stad. Or, even sleepier than Cape Town: Pringle Bay. Mandie's folks have a house there. Mike and I have taken our meds and done our homework, and I may or may not be pregnant. I don't have any symptoms (although you wouldn't, this early) apart from my skin that is breaking out from the meds.

My God, it's lovely to be out of Jo'burg and walking on the beach here, watching the churning of the sea. I stick my iPod on my arm and go for a run every morning. The place is bleached and windy and covered with fragrant *fynbos*. We spend the first few days unwinding: reading novels and newspapers, Pimm's-in-hand, napping on couches, going for long blustery walks with popped jacket collars.

We savour being away from traffic and deadlines and the general Jozi mania. In an unspoken agreement, we try to slow down time by moving languidly to make tea, or pour wine. We have long conversations and eat Indian vegetarian food. Nervous for the blood test, I dream of pregnancy and babies. There is tentative hope in every moment that I remember that this may be The Month.

Some Problem With the Connection

We drove into Cape Town today for the blood test. A part of me says, really? An hour's drive either way when I could just wait a couple of extra days to see if my shoulder starts hurting? But then I think those extra days would be torture and we may as well make a day of it.

The result took ages to come back. It was a terrible line, and I had to talk really loudly so that she could hear me. She had been calling and calling me, she said. There is some problem with the connection, she said. I said it's fine, it's fine. She said I must have tried to call you at least ten times. I'm sorry, I said, I don't know why you couldn't get through. I've been watching my phone like a hopped-up hawk. The calls weren't connecting, she said, as if that hadn't been immediately clear to me. I wanted to throttle her through the phone. Shut up, dreadful woman, I wanted to shout, I don't care about the fucking connection. I just want to hear the … and then, despite the static, I heard the word 'negative' clearly. When I heard her say it, I thought, of course it is. Why would I be pregnant? Why would this month be any different to the past 18 failed cycles? When I hung up, the other guys, stuck in the claustrophobic space with me as we were driving back to Pringle Bay, said kind and reassuring things, but the car was crowded with disappointment. I think they were waiting for me to cry, but I didn't.

...

I drank a lot of wine last night. It seems to be the only thing to do when you get a negative result on your 19th cycle (other than throwing yourself into the sea). I was trying to keep the atmosphere light, trying to let my hair down, trying to take advantage of the couple of days I have left before the pain arrives.

...

Bernadette (Mike's mom) called yesterday, saying that Cocoa hadn't been at home that day or the day before when she had popped in to feed them. We weren't too worried. We know cats (and especially our street-urchin cats) and how they do their own thing, visiting neighbours, taking impromptu naps on strangers' couches, etc. Mike and I keep telling each other that it's nothing to worry about, but neither of us are buying it. We're sure that if we cut our holiday short, the moment the plane touches down Cocoa will appear like the naughty little magical cat she is and jump on my lap. She's such an affectionate cat, I wonder if she's just staying at a neighbour's house for some attention while we're away. I know deep down that she would never run away. Some cats do, but Cocoa wouldn't.

...

I woke up this morning with a blooming sense of dread. For the first time, I think something bad has happened to Cocoa. Before, I was resisting flying back, resisting over-reacting, but I can feel now in my stomach that it's the right thing to do: I don't want to be in Pringle Bay anymore. I don't want to be anywhere but home now, looking for her.

I went for my regular early morning run but started crying halfway up a hill as that dreadful feeling surged inside me. It's like I started running not knowing if Cocoa was okay, and by the end of the run I knew she was not.

I wouldn't recommend bawling while you run up a hill. You can't get enough air, and you end up hyperventilating. You may or may not end up vomiting into the surrounding *fynbos* (and a little bit on your running shoes).

Come back, Cocoa, I say over and over in my head on our way home. Cat-coaxing. Come back.

Cocoa-less Day

We got back yesterday afternoon and spent the whole evening walking up and down our road, and the adjacent roads, calling Cocoa's name and shaking her bowl of food. Alex tried to help — he was pacing along with us and miaowing. Mike put up dozens of posters.

It was drizzling a bit and we were walking in the rain. I didn't care about getting wet but was worried that I wouldn't be able to hear her over the sound of the rain. Every now and then I would get that rush of dread and start crying, and her name would stick in my throat. I realise I must have looked like a completely insane woman, crying up and down the road in the rain, rattling a bowl of cat food.

She has a microchip so we have phoned every vet and SPCA we could think of. Surely, if we don't find her wandering the streets, we will find her this way? But no one has any news on the chip. They promise to call if she turns up.

After hours and hours of looking, it was dark and the rain was bucketing down, so we gave up the search for the day and went to bed. I have visions of her stuck somewhere, being doused in dirty rainwater. Hungry, or hurt. Hearing us calling her but not being able to escape.

I keep hoping she will somehow get the memo that we are back and come slinking in. I keep hoping that we'll wake up to a little black cat purring on our bed. But we woke up to another Cocoa-less day today.

She Was Still Warm

I couldn't stand not knowing what happened to my little Cocoa cat, I thought nothing could be worse, but this is worse. Our neighbour from across the street came back from Cape Town today and saw our posters. Called me, and told me what had happened. I sobbed on the phone. I didn't care what he thought. I bawled and thanked him, and then passed the phone to Mike so that he could finish the conversation. I knew she hadn't run away, I had known it all along.

The day before the neighbour left for holiday (just after we had left for Pringle Bay), he had an early morning stroll to the shop up the road, to buy a newspaper. In the ten minutes it took to buy the paper and walk back, a little black cat had crawled into the space between his security gate and his front door. He guessed that she had been hit by a car and had died a few minutes later. She was still warm.

Oh, how my heart broke. She was still warm.

He stressed that it had been a matter of minutes: in other words, she didn't suffer. I choose to believe that, even if it isn't true. How I wish I could have been with her in those last minutes, to hold her and comfort her and tell her how much I loved her and how much she meant to me. How I wish she hadn't been alone, and scared, and in pain. Not knowing it was our cat, he very kindly took her body to the SPCA. I don't know why they didn't scan her for a chip. It could have saved us 8 days of dread and heart-gnawing worry. Now there is just deep heartache.

I don't ever remember being this heartsore about anything. My poor, poor Cocoa. I can't believe you're gone.

I phoned my mom to tell her, and could hardly speak. She said that I must remember that Cocoa was a rescue cat, born on Rockey street and destined for a hard life, but because of us she had a wonderful life. It may have been short, but it was good, and full of love, and what else could any cat (or human) want? It made me cry more, but made me feel better.

RIP Cocoa. My short cat, my eternal kitten.

. . .

I still miss Cocoa every day. I miss her bottomless desire for affection. I miss her little body on my lap as I work, like she was a (furry) hot water bottle. I miss her feline intuition: how she would come to me when I was in pain and cuddle up and purr that huge trucking purr of hers, and make me feel better.

Alex misses her too. He hasn't settled down properly since she went missing and still calls for her every now and then, smashing our hearts every time. He had adopted her, and now she's gone. They would lie side by side, stretched out in the sun in the garden, or inside, on our bed. Sometimes in the exact same position. We all miss her. We give Alex a lot of extra attention, and that makes us all feel a bit better.

GOOD PRACTICE

We're starting another medicated cycle, the 2nd of a possible 3. This time I feel the side effects of the Femara: in a cruel twist it seems to have given me morning sickness. I had to write an exam today but felt so nauseous that I requested a table near the bathroom. I managed to keep the vom down for the two hours it took to write the exam, although I'm sure I missed out on a few marks while I sat there with my eyes closed, breathing slowly, trying to not lose my stomach on the shiny hall floor. I was pale (maybe green?) and my pen kept slipping out of my hand. The poor invigilator kept asking me if I was okay, patting my shoulder.

This is good practice, I kept telling myself. Soon I will really have morning sickness. Think of this as a rehearsal, I thought, as I gagged into the manky public toilet.

29

Stop the Fucking Bus

My brother, bless him, has just broken up with K, his latest live-in girlfriend. It wasn't that shocking. I could tell he wasn't that into her. The shocking thing came five minutes ago, when she called me to tell me that she's pregnant.

Stop the Fucking Bus, I thought.

Really, Universe? I've been broody since I was 12 and you give me a bum babymaker, but you give my brother — eternal bachelor who isn't interested in settling down — a fun accidental pregnancy with a woman he doesn't even like? I know, I know, not everything's about me, but fuck it, that's Not Cool.

30

Plot WIP

I think it's time to look at the plot again. This is where we were last time:

The Plot (Work In Progress)

1. Wedding! Honeymoon! Off the pill! So excited! Life is Awesome!

. . .

11. Baby-making situation looking a bit hopeless. Shoulder pain getting worse.

12. Start getting mightily attached to painkillers.

13. See psychologist to explain my woes. Psychologist makes me write this list.

14. BFG says sperm is monstrous. Try a round of turkey-baster AI. Negative.

15. Friend tells me to see her fertility specialist for a 2nd opinion. Enter: Dr G, AKA my hero.

16. Dr G turns diagnosis on its head. Sperm 100%. Surgery for me.

17. Have lap & hysteroscopy. Agony. Don't sleep for 4 days.

18. Shoulder pain returns. Uterus still stubbornly heart-shaped. Doubt Dr G.

19. Another surgery on uterus — successful. Slippy-slide of death is no more!

20. Fail PCT. Douche with common baking ingredient. Pass PCT.

21. Begin first of 3 medicated cycles. Negative.

22. Begin 2nd of 3 medicated cycles. Get faux morning sickness.

The world is spinning in my favour today: at my scan we saw that I have a 22mm follicle (the follicle is the thing that holds and releases the egg), which means that I'm just about to ovulate. I got to come off the awful Femara and get a trigger shot in my bum (okay, that sounded kinkier than it was), and we've got lots of homework to do over the next 48 hours.

Also: it's been a fantastic month for my business. I think it's a record. I'm working my arse off to get all the orders processed and dispatched. Boxes with Pulp stickers everywhere.

In other excellent news: Pin is coming home. After seven years in London, my BFF's back. My world today is a much better place.

31

Anything For A Story

E-e-e-e-e-e-e-e-k! A publisher has agreed to publish the novel I finished last year. It's called 'The Memory of Water' and is about a writer — not a very nice man — who will do anything for a story, including murdering the woman he loves. I have been happy-dancing and high-fiving all day. Just signed the contract. BEYOND excited.

How rewarding life can be, I tell myself. Look at my novels and notes and stories. Look at my florescent garden. Look how fertile I am in all ways but one.

BFN

Big Fucking Negative for our second medicated cycle. Not a surprise for anyone. I'm wondering why we're even trying these medicated cycles. They just make me feel sick and sore for half the cycle and disappointed for the other half.

I know the point of this journal is to write my feelings down to help to me process all these junk emotions, but I don't feel like it today. I don't feel like thinking about it.

...

The pain is smashing me. I'm on the floor and it just keeps kicking. I don't know what to do, but I can't do this anymore.

I'm not suicidal, but I do sometimes think that I would prefer to die than live like this.

32

Bad Lucky

South Africans have such a messed up idea of 'luck'.

I remember when my mom was hijacked the first time. Everyone told her how lucky she was. Lucky to be unharmed, lucky to be alive. She had a gun held to her temple and her car stolen — isn't she just the luckiest? She survived the second hijacking too, outside her recently deceased mother's house in Belgravia, telling her assailants that this time she would keep her handbag, thank you very much. And still, she breathes. What a lucky lady! The third time she decided she would keep her car, too. On a dark night in Melville, after my 21st birthday party, the bastards stopped their car in front of hers, sprang out, leaving their doors open, and knocked on her window with a gun. She put her foot down, and almost took their car door with her. Perhaps, that time, they were the lucky ones.

When our home was broken into recently, everyone's first reaction was : 'You are so lucky you weren't home!' and I have to stop my eyeballs from rolling back so hard that they spin out of my skull.

Recently people have also been saying how fortunate we are to have access to IVF. Don't get me wrong, I am extremely grateful that the technology exists, but no part of this journey has been 'lucky'. If anything it has been very bad-lucky indeed.

What is next? Telling people they're lucky to have a headache? Thank God for Panado, eh? At least it's not a brain tumour! What, you're actually undergoing chemo? Aren't you glad medicine is so advanced these days? And, look at the bright side, you don't need to shave your legs anymore! And save on the old hairdresser bill, eh? Awesome! What now? You say it's terminal? Now you get to shirk all your responsibilities and get cracking on that Bucket List! Travelling! Bungee jumping! While I have to sit at my desk! Your life is so exciting! You lucky, lucky fish. #blessed #doubleblessed

...

I've never been depressed before, so I wouldn't know how to recognise it, but I'm starting to wonder if I'm a little depressed. I'm wary of naming it, worried that if I create a label it might stick.

Before I was sad — sad about the (temporary) circumstances, sad about my Cocoa dying, sad about how I feel like things are working against me. But now it feels deeper than that, like it has moved past melancholy. Like the sadness is settling into my bones, and it won't be easy to shake, even if things get easier for me.

Micky alluded to it. It wasn't a diagnosis, not even a suggestion of a diagnosis: she just wondered out loud if I have been feeling depressed. I didn't know how to answer. Yes, I'm down — it would be weird not to be down in these circumstances — but depressed? I don't know. I haven't finished my degree in psychology yet. Isn't it her job, anyway, to decide?

So I did what I always do when I have a question that bothers me. I asked The Google.

If you type in 'Am I Depressed?' you'll get all the screening checklists you need to diagnose yourself. So here goes:

Over the last two weeks …

1. I have had little interest or pleasure in doing the things I usually enjoy — YES

2. I have felt down, depressed or hopeless — YES

3. I have had trouble falling or staying asleep, or I have been sleeping too much — YES

4. I have felt tired or have had little energy — YES

5. I have had a poor appetite or have been eating more than usual — NO, unless you count the extra chocolate and wine I've been consuming for self-medicating purposes.

6. I have felt bad about myself or felt that I am a failure or that I have let myself or family down — YES. Failure.

7. I have had trouble focusing on things — YES

8. I have been moving slower, or quicker, than usual — YES, moving (and thinking) in slow motion.

9. I have had thoughts that I would be better off dead or that I should hurt myself in some way — YES. Hurt myself: never. Better off dead: sometimes.

33

SISTERHOOD OF THE BROKEN BABYMAKERS

While asking Dr Google many questions over the last year or so I have come across various online infertility support groups. They are usually American or British. Once I used the phrase 'fall pregnant' on an American one and the women were amazed. What is this 'falling' you are speaking of? Apparently it makes it sound like an accident, something you succumb to, like falling ill. Of course, I thought, how un-American. Americans don't fall pregnant, they GET pregnant. They go out and get it. Booya.

As with any kind of online forum, the members have a vast amount of jargon acronyms that are specific to their plight.

IF, TTC, BD, DH, LO, IUI, ZIFT, GIFT, ICSI, POA, POAS. The first few times you try to decipher the posts is like decoding some sort of top secret communication.

Eventually I found the local support forum, called Fertilicare (FC). It has separate rooms for every spectrum of infertility: TTC (Trying To Conceive); Miscarriage / Loss; Rainbow Room (Gay couples); Secondary Infertility; Cigar Lounge (men's room); Adoption, etc. Basically, it's the Sisterhood of the Broken Babymakers.

I was used to the large American forums where there are hundreds of people posting, a lot of anonymity and not a great deal of ongoing relationships, so in my first post I just launched into a tirade about what an emotional mindfuck infertility can be. If I had hung around for a while, stalked the forum for a few days, I would have realised that it was proper etiquette to say hi and introduce myself before spattering my deepest angsty mess all over their wall.

Instead of slinging me out, or even mentioning my rudeness, the members left thoughtful and considered responses to my post. They made me feel welcome and comfortable immediately, despite my lack of manners. I soon learned that it's an intimate space, and everyone kind of knows each other, and quietly supports each other. For the first time since this nightmare started, I felt like I was not alone. Family and friends (and dear husbands) are one thing, but no one truly understands what it is like to be infertile until you are infertile yourself.

I think of when Pin was battling to conceive and how I (dismissively) said that she mustn't worry, that she would get pregnant, that I 'just knew she would'. I wouldn't dream of saying that to someone who is TTC now. I had to go through it myself to understand the nuances, and that there are no guarantees, no matter how many platitudes you spout. Telling someone that 'it will happen' is not helpful in the least.

There are never any harsh words on the forum, no judgement, just an open, mature place to share your experiences and ask advice from the more experienced members — the Veterans — and strictly no baby dust*.

*BD, or 'Baby Dust' is a mythical baby-powder-scented magical glitter that is enthusiastically and indiscriminately sprinkled, scattered, and flung around the American TTC forums. Like beach sand in your underwear, it gets everywhere, and is just as annoying. It may have a place in a newbie room when someone hasn't even been trying for six months, but offer a vet of four failed IVFs and two miscarriages a bit of baby dust and you'll be lucky to still have a head on your shoulders when that dust settles.

You can get to know the members by reading their signatures, which contain their IF history. My avatar is, fittingly, a heart and crossbones.

...

I've started to see everything in IVF currency. A weekend away? That's two injections of Menopur! Need to service your car? Uh-oh, that's going to cost you a vial of Cetrotide and a box of Uterogestan. New flatscreen? Out of the question. Rather keep the old tank you have perching precariously on an old wicker trunk in your lounge and get some tasty Intralipids instead. New car (with aircon!) — that would cost AT LEAST 2 full IVFs. Have you literally gone INSANE?

Also: I really think the fertility clinics are missing a trick by not selling vouchers for their drugs or treatments. I'd like nothing more than a few vouchers for ovulation drugs under the Christmas tree this year. In fact, every gift that is not a vial of something that will help me fall pregnant seems to be a miniature, gift-wrapped travesty.

34

50 Shades of Grey

I went on a shopping spree today. God knows I hate shopping. Can only abide it if I need something in particular and then I buy a whole lot of anything else I like in order to not have to repeat the process for as long as possible.

I feel about shopping the same way I feel about styling my hair. I have better things to do. I feel most comfortable in old jeans and a ponytail. I don't feel the need for lots of new things. I've been known to hang on to things until they're way past their best: my phone, my glasses, my MacBook, my car. The battery of my old laptop was literally falling out before I bought a new one. I'm not a slob — not always, anyway — I'm Low Maintenance.

I had been putting off this particular trip for as long as possible, but the time had come. I think the cashiers must think that I am either super-rich or that I have a shopping problem when they see how much I bring to the till. I always have the urge to tell them: It's not what you think. I only do this once or twice a year. It's actually less of a spree, and more of a marathon.

I hate the trying-on the most. Browsing the rails isn't too bad, it's when you have to muscle into the changing room with an armful of clothes that it starts to get iffy. Of course, the lighting is always terrible, everyone knows that. I'm sure it's been lamented for centuries. The stalls are stuffy, claustrophobic. Also: too many mirrors. It's not natural to be able to see your body from three different angles at once. You go in, fresh-faced, assured, with a healthy esteem, you leave pink and perspiring, with static Struwwelpeter hair, and bruised self-regard.

I got what I needed, plus an extra five shopping bags stuffed into my boot, after around three hours, which was good for me. Feeling triumphant, I missed the exit sign, and did an unintentional victory lap in the parking basement. On my return home, I paraded my new clothes in front of Mike, for our usual post-spree thumbs-up-thumbs-down ritual. There were a lot of thumbs-up. Feeling pleased with myself, I asked at the end: It was a good shop, wasn't it? And when he hesitated to reply, I demanded to know why. He said: It's all very nice. Good job.

But?! I demanded

But, he said, it's all grey.

It's not all grey! I insisted, looking for proof, and finding none. I only realised then that I had just bought a boot-full of grey clothes. They were nice clothes, and different shades, but they were all, unarguably, grey.

35

Xmas Ebola

I'm cursing these medicated cycles. I can't wait to see the back of them.

I don't know if it's the Femara making me ill, but bang on CD 12 of every cycle I have been sick. The first one wasn't too bad — I was green at the gills during my exam, I remember, and told myself it was good practice for morning sickness — but the second one was worse, like a mild food poisoning. This time it's full-blown stomach flu. I've been so-o-o-o-o sick.

It's Xmas eve, and I am wrapping last-minute presents. I hope I don't pass any of this special brand of dreaded lurgy on to my loved ones tomorrow.

I'm drinking Rehydrate, trying to hold it down. This kind of sickness always reminds me of a friend whose fiancé died. She told me the story years after it happened. I still feel such searing sorrow for her, I can't imagine the shock. He was ill with some kind of gastro, some kind of stomach bug, and she tried to keep him hydrated, fed him electrolytes, but she found him dead in the bathroom the next morning. A lovely, young, strong man. I'm not sure of the details, but I think the dehydration caused his heart to fail. The man she was in love with, the man she wanted to spend the rest of her life with. How do you get over something like that? She did. She's married now, has lovely kids. She has her happy ending.

Another friend lost her boyfriend in the Boxing Day Tsunami. They were together when the wave hit, when the warm salt-water and flotsam brimmed their room. He died in front of her. How can you continue to believe in God when something like that happens to you? She, too, has another life now, is happy and fulfilled.

What is the lesson? That there is a grand plan? Or that there is no plan at all? That we are all just mucking around in this messy life, vomiting and drowning, trying our best to grasp what we can?

I'll clinch Mike a little closer tonight, despite my diseased and pukey self. Sentimental, but it's Xmas eve, after all.

...

Still have my CD12 stomach flu (or reaction to Femara, or whatever it is), merry fucking Xmas. When I smell food, saliva rushes into my mouth, ready to splash into the toilet bowl (or someone else's car, or garden, if it catches me off-guard). I'm trying to get into the spirit but it's difficult when most of your attention is focused on trying to hold on to your stomach contents.

I was wondering if douching can make you sick like this. I know, it doesn't seem likely, but a lot of unlikely stuff has happened in the last few years. I Googled it, trying to find a link, but *nada*. So it is probably the drugs, or very bad luck. I've nicknamed it my Xmas Ebola, and spent the evening clutching my glass of sparkling water and *knyping*.

Being sick (and sober) on Xmas is bleak, but I'm more worried about tomorrow. We're driving to Port Elizabeth to visit Jack, Mike's grandfather (Chris's dad). He hasn't been well, and it's his (last?) birthday, so we're all driving down *en masse*. Usually it's around a ten-hour car trip. Aargh. Please let me be better tomorrow, or it may be the worst road trip ever.

...

May Jesus, Mary and Joseph bless the hungover elves of Boxing Day today. I managed the trip without expelling any bodily fluids on anything (or anyone), and can now, on holiday, finally stop *knyping*. The weather here is terrible, which is wonderful — all the more reason to cuddle up with chocolate and red wine and the new season of Top Chef Desserts.

...

I started bleeding today. CD15 — which is nine days early. At first I thought it may be implantation bleeding and almost fainted with excitement, but then there was too much blood. A crimson puddle of anti-joy. I'm usually super-regular so I don't know what's going on.

Perhaps the Xmas Ebola brought it on? Is that even possible? It might just be my continuing streak of bad luck, or the triumph of Murphy's Law. You know, the rule that if you wash your car it will rain? I was wearing my white bikini, which is kind of the same thing.

LATE

So after bleeding mid-cycle, my period is now four days late. LATE! I'm never late. Dare I hope? Dare I hope that we managed to conceive the month before we were due to start IVF? In the third of three medicated cycles?

Wouldn't it be hilarious if I did actually fall pregnant on holiday? It would add to the infuriating urban legend that going on vacay can cure even the most stubborn case of infertility.

My heart is jumping around in my chest like it knows something that I don't. Our appointment with Dr G is in three days' time. If I don't come on by tomorrow, and don't have any shoulder pain, I'll go for a blood test. Eeeeeeeeeeeek!

BLUE SPARK

When there was still no sign of Aunt Flow this morning, at five days late, I went for a blood test. If I had just waited another hour I would have saved myself a trip to the lab and 200 bucks. The moment, the very moment, I got home, I felt a blue spark in my shoulder, and I knew.

The third cycle had been a bust.

Bring Out The Big Guns

So after months and months of tossing the idea of IVF in the air — with neither of us really wanting to touch it — we seem to have all of a sudden grown balls. A pair of giant, hairy, balls.

It's been almost 2 years. We're tired of the failed cycles, we're sick to death of the pain. Dr G has said it's now or never. It's time, as Mike puts it, to bring out the Big Guns.

I'm nervous/excited. Are we really going to do this?

36

IVF #1

This is the IVF deal with Dr G:

1. We'll do short protocol with intralipids.

2. Stim hard because of my ancient ovaries. We're talking 5 amps of Menopur a day instead of the usual 3.

3. Hoping for 8 – 12 eggs. Less than 8 means we won't have a lot to work with. More than 12 may indicate bad quality eggs. Less is less, more is less. We need 10, more or less.

4. Will aim to transfer 2 embryos on day 3 or 5.

5. Estimated date of transfer will be first week of Feb. (That means I may HAVE A BABY IN MY ARMS BY NEXT XMAS.)

6. He gave us the (what seem like excellent) odds of 52% chance of achieving pregnancy.

7. 15 – 30% chance of twins! Eek!

8. We have to sell all our possessions to afford it. We don't care. Okay, we care a little bit.

9. Hope the twins won't mind living in a homeless shelter.

10. I'm not sure why this is still a list.

11. I'll stop now.

Mike pressed the doc on the chance of us having twins. Before it seemed like a terrifying result, now we're getting so desperate it seems like an excellent deal: pay for one IVF, get two babies. Dr G said: 'Listen here. We cater for the needy, not the greedy.'

...

It occurred to me today that I have had more people looking at my golden goose in one month during fertility treatment then I have had lovers my entire life. The first few times a new doc used a dildo cam on me I had the urge to joke — entirely inappropriately — that they could have at least bought me dinner first.

I hear that it is good practice for giving birth. Apparently whatever hint of modesty you have around your nethers is completely stripped as you head into advanced labour. You lie there, legs spread under the bright lights while every gynae, nurse, midwife, doula, anaesthetist, paediatrician and sandwich-trolley man looks on.

Sometimes one of them comes closer to get a better look, perhaps sticks a few fingers in to measure your cervix dilation. Your eyes are closed: you just hope that it wasn't the sandwich-trolley man.

INTRALIPIDS

The girls on the internet forum keep bringing up intralipids, wondering whether they work or not.

Intralipids are basically the way you feed a patient who can't eat or use a feeding tube: a soya-based high fat, high protein emulsion (yum!) administered intravenously. It's an expensive three-hour process that can make you feel sick. The idea is not immediately appealing. I know what you're thinking: can't you just eat a cupcake, and some crispy bacon? Why do you have to get nurses and latex gloves and needles involved? That, I'm afraid, will remain one of life's bigger mysteries.

The theory is (and it sounds like it really is just a theory) that the intralipids somehow calm the mercenaries in your blood, or the natural killer cells. In some women who battle to fall pregnant, the NK cells are overly aggressive and successfully target any foreign matter like snipers on speed. The problem is that they can't always tell the difference between unwanted matter (viruses, bacteria, tie-dyed shirts) so they just keep their fingers on the trigger and sorry for you if you're a hopeful little just-burrowed embryo.

I asked Dr G if he thought it was a good idea. He

was surprised that I knew about it — he has no idea how much we gossip on the forum — and said we may as well try it. He isn't entirely convinced of the results but is keen to try anything that shows a positive correlation. It's expensive for something that no one is really sure works, but our reasoning is that if you're already spending ten times the amount on IVF, best you do anything you can to up your chances of it working. Who knows what the tipping point will be?

He agrees that we should do anything we can to make it work. He described our situation as walking on a tightrope, which made me suitably anxious. I think he thinks there is hope, but not much. We need to grab this chance and give it everything we've got.

ORANGE THOUGHTS

My acupuncturist wants me to go on this crazy diet before IVF. No hormones (i.e. meat or dairy), no allergens (grains of any kind), no processed food, no sugar, caffeine or alcohol. If you, like me, count caffeine and alcohol as their own individual food groups, you'll see that there is not a lot left to consume. Limited fruit, and no carbs after 4pm. Eight glasses of water a day. Mike makes me a smoothie every morning, which is a good start. I have no idea what I will eat for the rest of the day. I picture myself squirrelling away berries and nuts, like Scrat on Ice Age.

It makes sense to me not to have any junk in your body when you start IVF. You want to be as healthy and non-toxic as possible. I have to do everything I can to make this IVF work.

Here is my plan:

1. No running; yoga is okay.

2. No booze.

3. No coffee. No, not even decaf. No Ceylon.

4. Commit to every session with acupuncturist and don't cancel due to workload.

5. Try the squirrel/monkey diet (i.e. eat only vegetable matter).

6. ABC: Always Be Cool.

7. Think positive, orange thoughts (orange is the Chinese colour of fertility).

8. Listen to the fertility meditation / hypnotherapy track as often as possible.

9. Keep an open mind.

10. Trust in the universe (even though she can be a total bitch).

11. Intralipids.

12. Remember that everything is as it should be, which is different to believing in 'Fate'. No one truly believes in fate. Ask a fatalist if they look for cars before crossing the road and I bet you they'll say yes.

...

We had Chris over for dinner last night. I was telling him all the things I was going to do, to make sure that this IVF works. He said that the rate I'm going, we'll put back 2 embryos and get triplets.

Not Tonight, Honey, My Babymaker Has a Headache

I find it distinctly UNfunny that you are not allowed to have sex during the month of IVF. It feels weird and wrong. If I get pregnant I'll be kind of like Jesus's mom. Immaculate Conception. I'm not strictly speaking a virgin (I'll hazard a guess that she wasn't, either) but it will be miraculous nonetheless.

IVF duties: Him vs. Her

What Women Have To Do

1. Have period, count cycle days, make appropriate appointments.

2. Go for scans at the crack of dawn's bum.

3. Basically give up their modesty of the VJJ variety.

4. Give up booze and sex.

5. Have blood tests and three-hour long doses of intralipids.

6. Have loads of injections to stimulate ovulation.

7. Suffer from ovarian hyperstimulation syndrome if too stimulated.

8. Be judged if not stimulated enough (i.e. labelled a 'poor responder').

9. Have more scans to monitor follicle maturation.

10. Have more blood tests.

11. Get Cetrotide shots to hold off ovulation.

12. Get trigger shot to trigger ovulation.

13. Go under anaesthetic for egg recovery (like organ harvesting, but think caviar instead of liver or lung).

14. Field the embryologists calls with heart-in-throat.

15. Field all the friends' and relatives' questions with positive updates.

16. Have more intralipids.

17. Have more scans.

18. Have more blood tests.

19. Have the embryos transferred to uterus.

20. Have more intralipids.

21. Take oestrogen pills and progesterone pessaries (pessa-what-what?) a hundred times a day.

22. Wait two agonising weeks.

23. Go insane, analysing every twitch and twinge.

24. Pee on too many sticks.

25. Curse the sticks and throw them all away.

26. Go for more blood tests.

27. Wait for more agonising hours while the lab takes their sweet time to get back to you.

28. Field the call of the lab person, trying not to weep/shout for joy into the phone.

29. Let Everyone know the result.

30. BFN? Repeat steps 1 − 29.

31. BFP? Have another blood test the day after, and the day after that, to make sure that beta is doubling, to confirm that the pregnancy is viable.

32. Then the real work begins.

What Men Have To Do

1. Wank.

The Wounded Receptionist

We've started! We've started! Scan this morning at 6am and blood tests were a go. I have my purple bag and it's full of vials and needles and alcohol patches.

Everyone who does IVF at VL has a purple zip-up bag. You get it when you buy all your meds, a free gift, like a complimentary lipstick in a shade you'd never buy. You imagine having a bumper sticker on the bag saying: 'I spent R50K on IVF and all I got was this crappy purple cooler bag.'

Once you have your bag you notice other people with their bags. Some look brand-new, like mine, others are scuffed, like they have been kicked around the room a few times. When you see someone else with a purple bag you smile at them in what you think is a supportive way. The ones that snark back at you are the Vets. They know there is no place for sunshiny optimism. They've already pissed away their pension plan, the hope of a new car and a few holidays in Bali, now they are just there to get on with it, and all these fresh-faced newbies are in their way. Despite getting there for your scan at 5:30am you inevitably have to wait an hour or two to get scanned, because there are 20 people there before you. It's like trying to get into a NYC club, just with different bouncers, and different drugs. Vets should get a preferential queue, like the 10-items-or-less till at Pick 'n Pay.

Usually Mike and I sit frowning at our laptops, smashing our keyboards, and getting as much work done as we can while we wait. I can imagine people looking at us and thinking: No wonder they can't conceive, they've practically got 'Type-A' stamped on their foreheads. I let Mike off today so it's just me and my trusty computer, which I set up at a really handy desk in the entrance of the room they do procedures in. The only problem was that every second person who came in asked me questions I didn't know the answers to, like where to make their 'deposit'. Despite being hooked up to an IV, I apparently looked like a receptionist. One of the nurses laughed about it and called me 'The Wounded Receptionist'.

The intralipids are really cold, and it can be uncomfortable, so you put a hot water bottle on your arm as it's going in and that makes it feel better. Thank God I took my machine and was able to work there or I would be stressing out. The whole palaver took SEVEN HOURS. And no complimentary tea and rusks for me — I'm on the monkey diet!

It's only day 1 and I've already had enough of needles. Today I had the Menopur shot, bloods drawn, an IV, and acupuncture. I know it's just the beginning. I'm going to look like a heroin addict soon. Or a colander.

Poison

5 amps of Menopur a day is too much for my body to handle. The pain in my shoulder has spread, poisoning my arm all the way down to my wrist, and freezing my ribs. The whole right side of my body feels cracked open. It's hard to breathe. No sleep.

The pain is worst when I lie down. I tried sleeping

sitting up in bed and got a few hours. Am worried that either the painkillers or the pain (or both) will be toxic to my babymaker. If I was an embryo I wouldn't choose this hell chamber as a host.

37

MAN'S SEARCH FOR MEANING

I'm trying to live 'in the moment', and not worry too much about what the future holds, but what about when The Moment is filled with pain? Chris bought me a copy of Victor Frankl's 'Man's Search for Meaning' and I got so much out of it that I read it again immediately, to cement the ideas in my head. His idea resonated with me: that to live a good and satisfying life you have to find meaning in your suffering. There is always suffering, but it's up to you to convert it to good. My problem is that I can't see the meaning. I don't know why I'm going through this. Perhaps it will become clear to me later. If I can't find meaning, maybe I have to make meaning, but I don't really know how to start with that, either.

...

Our scan today showed that we have around seven follicles. It's good. Not great, but good. All seven are on my dodgy right ovary (which Mike calls my 'smoker's ovary').

The left ovary was nowhere to be seen. I think he was shy because he knows he's in trouble. Lazy-ass ovary.

Doc: 'Oh, look, 7 follies on the right. Excellent. Now let's have a look at the ... hold on.'

Lazy-ass ovary: *hides*

Doc: 'What the? Er ... We seem to have lost your left ovary.'

Seven follicles is enough to go ahead with the program. We are relieved, and tentatively excited. I told the doc that the stims are killing my shoulder. He shrugged sympathetically and offered me more Synap, which I jumped at, despite it not really making a dent in the stimming pain. At schedule 5 it's stronger than anything else I have. I told him I'm worried that the pain will make my body a sub-optimal environment for the embryo, but he's not concerned. Maybe it's because he doesn't know how bad it is.

On the way out he said to me: 'Don't forget to bring your left ovary in for your next scan.'

...

I would kill for sleep. Just a few hours to escape this pain. God Almighty I feel like throwing myself off a bridge.

An Orange a Day

My lovely Pin is sending me pictures of an orange thing every day. Today it was baby Ben's butternut-smeared mouth. Yesterday, an autumn leaf.

. . .

In a pain-fevered sleep last night I dreamt that Mike had an affair and that his mistress was pregnant. She was a blank slate: she had no face, just a belly ballooning under a pretty summer dress. They were going to have a baby, he shrugged, he'd have to leave me. He had responsibilities now. Could I blame him?

I may or may not have kicked him under the covers. Bastard. It took a while to forgive him his imagined betrayal.

THE SYNAP FORTÉ FAN CLUB

Roela brought over some extra painkillers for me today. She broke her wrist really badly a few months ago playing netball and was living on Synap, and we exchanged Synap stories. We know it is not good for us but we don't care. The Synap Forté Fan Club. Her arm has healed now (with the help of some bad-ass titanium plates and screws) and she has some pills left over. I almost kissed her. We had tea and chatted while she glowed in all her Fairy-Godmother-of-Pain-Relief Glory.

. . .

I told the acupuncturist that the stims are making me so sore I could vomit. She tried this weird thing on me called Chinese 'cupping'. It sounds vaguely sexual, I know, but she's not that kind of girl (I don't think) (I may be wrong).

Cupping has been around since 300 AD. It's supposed to be 'the opposite of massage' and I agree: Massage is usually a pleasant experience. The negative pressure is supposed to loosen muscles, improve blood flow, and sedate the nervous system. She took these glass cups and put them on my skin, then lit something on them to cause a vacuum. She did around six, including one on each shoulder. The suction is intense, pulling your skin into mounds, and leaving huge hickies after the glass is removed, which take days to fade into bruises. My mom was horrified. Even though the cupping didn't work, I liked having the outward show of injury. It felt right.

38

6 Eggs

Today I went in for the egg recovery. That's when they stick a long needle up your Aunt Betty and poke around for goodies using an ultrasound. A bit like those old dry-handed guys on the beach with nicotine-stained moustaches and metal detectors.

EGG RECOVERY. I've been looking forward to it for days. Four golden syllables: an-aes-the-tic. It was beautiful and delicious. I was so grateful to be knocked out that apparently I kept thanking the nurses when I was coming to. There was a sticker on my hand saying: '6 eggs', with a smiley-face. Half a dozen eggs.

6 is a lovely number, just look at it! It looks pregnant.

...

All this talk of eggs has made me think of that silly 'Two Ronnies' skit when they talk in letters of the alphabet.

Mike does it in an especially funny accent.

F U N E X? (Have you any eggs?)

...

The embryologist phoned and gave me excellent news. We have a 100% fertilisation rate! It is uncommon. I'm so relieved. I have in the past wondered if our guys just don't like each other, but apparently they like each other very much indeed. Wooo hoo! This makes me really happy. One of the eggs was immature (How could the embryologist tell? Was he pulling faces? Blowing raspberries? Grow up, egg! What are you, 4?! Act your age please, not your shoe size), but of the five mature eggs all were fertilised, so as I write this we have five little embryos. Incredible! There they are sitting in their little glass dishes at VL, summoning the courage to split their cells and grow. I wish I could see them, kiss their lids, tell them that I am waiting for them.

...

Three of the five embryos are growing well, two stalled at the starting gate, stopping at day 3.

Three embryos is good. Three is enough. As the girls on the forum say: it only takes one. I know waiting till day 5 is best, but I wish I had them inside me now, instead of lying in a glass dish in a lab. Our embryos! Alive and waiting for transfer.

May They Be Cling-ons

Transfer day.

We made it to day 5, and had three viable embryos. Two goodies, and one dodgy-looking one that only a mother could love. The doc showed us pictures of the blastocytes and I wanted to frame them and hug them to my chest, like I did in the hobbit-warren fertility cave. Oh, my little blasts, my little babies, I was thinking, like the crazed woman I have become. Come to mama. Come on board the mothership.

The nurse takes a photo as the embryos are inserted: there is a small, hopeful flash of light as it happens, like a shooting star. I haven't let go of the print-out since she put it in my clammy paw.

We decided, under the doc's guidance, to put back the two healthy-looking embryos. Lawrence Twins here we come! While I was sad to lose the other three (YES I WANTED ALL FIVE), I'm deliriously happy and hopeful to have two actual embryos inside me right now. I mean, I'm virtually pregnant, aren't I?

I think two is a great number, two babies would be an absolute blessing. Tough going, sure, but imagine the sheer wonder. The joy. Double the happiness. Twins went from being an unwelcome result to, perhaps, the best result possible. I know I'm gushing. Next thing I'll be addicted to fertility treatments like Octomom. There is also always the chance of accidental multiples: there have been stories of freakishly enthusiastic embryos splitting in utero, one couple undergoing IVF put two embryos back and got six babies. I'll stick to the dream of twins, for now.

Mandie and Avish gave me some orange undies to wear today, to seal the deal. If this works I will keep them forever.

Bernadette is burning a candle for us.

Pin sent me a pic of cookie cutters spelling out 'New Home' and a note that almost made me cry.

Melissa emailed me, wishing me luck. She said: 'I can't believe you have babies inside you! May they be 'Clingons' in the Mothership.'

I thought the two-week wait would be the most difficult thing about this process, but it's plain sailing compared to the stimming. The pain has all but vanished and there are no more jabs. We've done everything we can. I keep my days as stress-free as possible. I meditate and listen to my fertility hypnosis track. I risk being mistaken for a Hare Krishna because of all the orange I wear. I wake up every morning and think: I have two babies inside me. At night I put my hands over my babymaker and send the twins warm, welcoming energy. I'll be such a good mother to them. Please God let them implant. Please God let me be pregnant. Please God give me my Big Fat Positive.

I told Mike that I hope we have twins so that we can get those cute onesies: the one says 'COPY' and the other one says 'PASTE.'

...

One of the pills I have to take this IVF cycle,

Ecotrin, comes in a child-proof container.

A ha ha ha ha ha ha ha.

Letting Go

Sometimes this whole infertility Fuck Circus seems like a giant lesson in letting go. I'm a self-confessed control freak: not exactly anal, not OCD, but I like things a certain way. More than anything, I like to have control over the things that are important to me. And I like to get my own way. With IVF it's out of my hands. In a way that drives me crazy, but in another way it's a relief. When I start feeling anxious about our test day I try to stop and breathe, and remember that I have done everything I can. The rest is up to science and luck.

...

This morning, while making our ritualistic Sunday breakfast, I broke the first egg into the frying pan and gasped.

'Bubs!' I said. (I call Mike 'Bubs', I've never been sure why.) He came over and stared at the hot pan, too. There were two yolks. One egg. Two yolks.

'Hee!' I shrilled, crazy-eyed, doing an impromptu (and not very co-ordinated) tap dance. 'Twins!'

Mike looked pleased.

I broke the next one. It also had two yolks. Two sets of twins. WTF?

Mike looked slightly less pleased.

...

Today I inspected my naked body in the full-length mirror, trying to find some kind of hint of pregnancy. My stomach has never been flat, so that's a red herring, right there. I scrutinised my breasts. Felt them for tenderness (none), or Montgomeries* (none).

*Montgomeries are the little bumps you get on your nipple when you are preggo. They are glands that help your little baby find your boob with his eyes shut from metres away in a crowded room, like an especially proficient sniffer dog. (In my imagination the dog is a Pointer named, of course, Montgomery).

Peeing On A Stick

Most infertile women have an extremely unhealthy relationship with home pregnancy tests, also known on the forum as Evil Sticks. Taking a test is called POAS: Peeing On A Stick, as in: My period is an hour late so I'm going to POAS. They are referred to as evil because of their inaccuracy and their sheer addictiveness. You may have track-marks from shooting up Cetrotide in the public toilet at gym but evil sticks are the crack cocaine of the infertile community. We buy them by the hundreds and use them by the handful. We pay in cash and hide the receipts from our partners. If no second line shows up on the first test it is binned as a dud, and a further two are used to confirm the Big Fat Negative. If there is a special on sticks at Dischem you'll know about it before the shop assistants do, courtesy of the support forum.

We urge our friends on the forum to not POAS. It is almost always a bad idea. It is not worth the uncertainty, and the heartache. We know the monkey on your back on a first-name basis (Frederick), because we have the same monkey on ours. We ardently urge our forum sisters to not POAS while typing with one hand, because we are, ourselves, at that exact moment, peeing on a stick.

I am in fact the exception to this habit, not out of choice or willpower, but because of the bloody windrose I have pinned inside my shoulder. Before I can even get the box out of the bathroom cupboard on CD28 my diaphragm is spelling out 'No Dice' in morse code down my ribcage, like bloody Frederick on a xylophone.

The two sticks I have are almost three years old, bought when I turned 30 and started trying-not-trying. They have been relinquished to a dark corner in the bathroom cupboard. I picture them sad, and gathering dust. They give new meaning to the phrase 'On The Shelf'.

SOME PEOPLE HAVE ALL THE LUCK

As our blood test appears on the horizon and we tiptoe tentatively towards it ('What if it worked? Eek! What if it's twins? Double-eek! Happy-dance. Nervous-dance. High-fives all round) we try to stay positive and keep our nerve.

Mike: 'How do you feel?'

Me: 'Fine. You?'

Mike: 'No, I mean, how do you FEEL-feel?'

Me: 'Normal.'

Mike: 'Not pregnant?'

Me: 'I don't know. I've never been pregnant!'

Mike: 'Hungry?'

Me: 'Always!'

Mike: 'So then you don't feel different?'

Me: 'No.'

Mike: 'Oh.'

Me: 'Wanna feel them?'

Mike: 'What?'

Me: 'My boobs.'

Mike: 'Why?'

Me: 'You need a reason?'

Mike: 'Do they feel different?'

Me: 'I don't think so.'

Mike: 'Oh.'

Me: 'That doesn't mean I'm not pregnant! Haven't you seen that show "I Didn't Know I Was Pregnant".

Mike: 'Huh?'

Me: 'It's always, like, a teenager with a flat stomach and irregular periods who starts getting stomach pains and they rush her to the ER. She thinks it must be the dodgy Mexican food she ate the day before with the boyfriend she swears she's not having sex with but then ends up giving birth in the car on the way to hospital.'

Mike: 'Kaiser Soze!'

Me: 'And then she's all, like, "I don't know how it happened!" as if no-one ever told her that if you have unprotected sex in Mexican restaurants you can fall pregnant. Especially when you're young and super-fertile. "Boo! Poor me! It was only that one time! He bought me nachos!! Now I have this baby."'

Mike: 'Unbelievable.'

Me: 'Yip. Some people have all the luck!'

...

Can't sleep.

Not because I'm in pain, not this time, but because I'm days away from a pregnancy test that may change my life. The thought that I may be pregnant — or rather, the question: 'Am I pregnant?' — loops around in my head until it is battered, like a bird trapped in a conservatory.

Or: a canary the colour of a lemon that I've sent down the mineshaft: the vortex of infertility. Will it come up alive? Or will its little black eyes be glazed over and dull in death? Will my observing it (read: obsessing over it) change the outcome? It will, if you believe in quantum physics. Schrödinger's Budgie — eaten by his cat while no one was watching.

...

Holy Moses this waiting is TORTURE. I wish we were on holiday somewhere away from this low grade fever, this burning tension. Mere days to go until we know. You'd think that we've waited so long, what is an extra couple of days? But every hour stretches out in front of me like a rubber band, threatening to snap.

...

One more night of restlessness, one more day to dream. Dear God please, please, PLEASE can I be pregnant.

I lie prostrate on the floor, begging any deity that will listen: This is a rare chance, I tell them, I've done everything I can. Please tip the odds in my favour.

...

The citrus-coloured canary appears to be dead. The rubber band has snapped. The fire has started in my shoulder.

39

My Bloody Compass

There's no point in going for the blood test, although VL is insisting. My shoulder flared up last night. It started with a subtle knock-knock-knocking of pain, which I tried to ignore. Told myself I was imagining it. Then it got worse, quickly, as if to convince me, and I had to accept that the IVF didn't work. I didn't even get the chance to pee on a stick, which would have been a nice touch. It would have brought the saying 'Pissing away money' to life. So much money. So much hope. So many hours of treatment and dreaming of a better life. The life I was meant to live. So I went for the stupid test and of course it was a Big Fat Negative. My divining rod of a shoulder, my bloody compass, is never wrong.

I'm heartbroken.

My eyes are swollen. I feel as if someone has died. I was so positive this cycle. I did absolutely everything I could and everything went well. Everything went well up until, I guess, it didn't.

I'm trying to not take it personally — although I'm not sure it gets any more personal than this — and I'm trying to have perspective. I'm trying to convince myself that just because this one didn't work, it doesn't mean that it will never happen. But some kind of devastating knowledge is weighing down on me, a feeling that it will never happen. It's crushing me.

If we had loads of money and loads of time, this news wouldn't be as devastating as it is. We could keep trying until something, somewhere in the universe or inside my body, clicks. But we're not in that position. I curse myself for not becoming a CA. Accountants make shedloads of money. Why did I have to "follow my passion" to sell books and write stories? Do you realise how many books you need to sell to afford just one amp of Menopur?

But even if we manage to beg, borrow and steal more cash, the more worrying thing is the question of it working. My babymaker is busted. I tried to fix it but, like a post-accident panel-beaten car, no matter how much time, money and love you spend on it, it will never be 100% again.

I'm sitting on the lounge floor trying to work. Trying to get on with the day. I have the TV on in the background for maximal distraction, otherwise I play Imogen Heap over and over and cry so hard that I can't see my screen. Laila the new kitten is cuddled up on my lap. An email comes through — an invitation to K's baby shower. A thing with a teddy bear and blue ribbons and something about a baby boy bringing joy and I know that this time I won't be able to go, despite him being my first and only nephew. Until further notice, my Brave Face is lying at the bottom of an ocean somewhere. Cool and dark. Sleeping with the fishes. I wouldn't mind being there too.

...

I need to know why it didn't work. On a scientific level and on a spiritual level. I hate that there are no answers.

I wish that we hadn't gone all out with this cycle. If we had held something back we could have changed something for the next try. Added something to the mix, if for no other reason than to give us hope. It will be very difficult to do another cycle without hope.

...

My Facebook status today:

Life can be tough, but it doesn't mean you should harden your heart.

...

It was a difficult weekend. Mike and I avoided everyone and embarked on a massive Campaign of Distraction to keep our minds (and hearts) off our infertility. Denial and distraction were our friends.

Simon said to Mike: 'The answer isn't NO, it's just NOT NOW' (He's in sales).

If only that were true. If that were true we wouldn't be grieving. If there was some way I could magically see into the future and glimpse a child of ours, this journey would be a piece of cake. We would go through the motions until we finally get to pass GO and collect our baby (and our 100 rand).

It's the not knowing that makes it difficult. It's the Not Having a Fucking Clue.

KARMIC JOKE

Sometimes I think that my infertility is a punishment for being selfish. To teach me a lesson. It sounds paranoid, I know. Maybe it's natural to look for reasons when it feels like the universe is against you.

I know that I am self-absorbed. Now more so than ever. I'm not saying that I've never been kind, or generous, or that I'm a bad person. Just that my main priority is usually ... me. I think of others, but usually I think of myself first.

The very act of having your own biological kids is inherently selfish, isn't it? I mean, I know parenting is mostly selfless, and requires constant sacrifice, but deciding to have your own — it satisfies a biological need — no one else's biological need but your own. The earth certainly doesn't need more humans, schools don't need more children.

But I wonder if it's more personal than that. I wonder if it is, in particular, about me breaking up with a beloved ex-boyfriend because I found someone else who I thought would make a better father. In real life it was a lot more complicated than that. I was very much in love with B. I loved him truly and furiously as you do your first love. I gave him everything I had to give. We lived together for four years and I adored his family. I remember telling my father that he was The One. On a snowy night in Switzerland we looked at engagement rings in shop windows. Something happened that broke the relationship, and even though I was willing to stay and make it work — and did, for a long time — it snapped me out of my mesmerism. He didn't want kids, but would have them because I wanted them so much. Perhaps, I remember thinking, that's not the ideal way to begin a family. I saw myself ten years down the line, divorced with two kids, like my mother was, and wondering what the fuck I had been thinking, having kids with a man who didn't want them in the first place.

And then, without me even looking for him, Mike was in front of me. Suspiciously handsome, understatedly sexy, funny. From the beginning our relationship was intense in every way. I don't believe in love at first sight, but I spotted his soul the first minute we spoke. I sat across from him and thought: we'll get on. Everyone else at the table disappeared. We exchanged boarding school horror stories, mostly about hostel food. He told me about someone finding an animal tooth in their casserole, and I told him about my theory that they used to grind up whole chickens for our chicken pies, the parts we used to find in there. He told me about mother-of-pearl-shiny beef, I told him about getting yellow curry on blue plates, resulting in a nauseous neon green sauce.

We had other things in common, too. We were the same age, both in advertising, working in the same agency. We both liked travelling, photography, architecture, property investment, red wine and Dave Matthews. We both wanted children. We connected, we hit it off. Completely and irreversibly. When I left that day, I thought: Uh Oh.

In a way, Mike was eerily similar to B. Both were the eldest of three boys, both boarding school grads, both of UK descent and lovely families. Both, it goes without saying, clearly have incredible taste when it comes to women.

It turned out to be messy. I don't usually 'do' drama in relationships but this time I had no choice. I had to make a decision that would alter the course of my life. I didn't cheat on B, not physically, anyway. I broke up with him as soon as I realised that I was in love with Mike, a relationship that was yet to be consummated by even a kiss. I broke up with B, still loving him, knowing that Mike was due to leave for London, to work there.

I cried for days. It was the most difficult thing I had ever done (until now). To make it worse, I couldn't tell B the truth. I didn't have the courage, and I didn't want him to know that I had chosen someone else over him. I was a coward, and I reasoned that I had done enough damage.

Mike moved away, Mike moved back. He turned out to be the love of my life. We bought a house, adopted two cats, and lived happily ever after. Until now.

Now Karma's tapping me on the shoulder.

Karma: (tap tap tap)

Me: 'Do you mind? That's my sore shoulder. Your doing, no doubt.'

Karma: 'Remember that time you left someone, breaking his heart?'

Me: 'It was the right thing to do. It broke my heart, too.'

Karma: 'The right thing for *you*.'

Me: 'Yes, the right thing for me. And my unborn children.'

Karma: 'Ah, well now,' (snickers) 'it looks like the joke's on you.'

Have you ever known a Karmic joke to be funny? *Kak* sense of humour, that Karma.

40

Rebound IVF

Clinic B is having a Valentine's Special — they are offering IVF at half-price for the month of February. Mike and I are going to visit, if for no other reason than a 2nd (3rd? 4th? 17th?) opinion. Although they are a more affordable clinic, they have an excellent reputation. Maybe they will pick up something that VL missed. Maybe we'll just jump right into a special-price-just-for-you discount-discount IVF.

Heartbroken? BFNs getting you down? Try rebound IVF!

Or, as Rollo May (slightly more eloquently) puts it, "The capacity to move ahead in spite of despair."

...

The Clinic B doctors seem very nice. Knowledgeable, caring, down-to-earth, and they did indeed give us an alternative opinion, but not one that we were happy to hear. While Dr G thinks we should do another round of IVF as soon as possible, Clinic B thinks that until my endo is dealt with (again) there is little hope of conceiving. Endo creates a toxic environment, and they don't see the point in investing in an IVF cycle until it's cleared up. They scanned me and found a large cyst on my ovary — and said no way they would stim me when it looks like a battleground down there. I was so disheartened to see that damn cyst. Fucking endo. Fucking fuck.

Their advice is way different to VL's. They recommend I have another lap (it's only been 6 months since my last one) and/or go on a drug called Zoladex to shut down the endo (in fact it shuts down the babymaker, full stop). That creaking you hear? That's the 'CLOSED' sign swinging in the breeze. Zoladex basically puts you into early menopause. It seems to be a drastic step. If I trip over something (Laila!) I don't want to have to worry about falling and breaking a hip. I don't want granny bones at 32 or tumbleweeds in my babymaker.

...

I was born stubborn. Some people would say that it's because my star sign is Taurus (bull). My mother would tell you that I, like her, could out-mule a mule. When I was a toddler I decided that I no longer liked my crèche. Because I wasn't good at communicating (I only spoke Monkey) it took a while for my mom to get the message. One morning she put me in the back seat and before she could reach her car door I jumped up and locked all the doors from the inside, locking her out. It took half an hour of pleading and a promise from her that I wouldn't have to go to the dreaded crèche before I would open her door for her. I spent the rest of the day as a kindergarten refugee, hiding under her desk at school, being fed scrap paper and crayons, and the occasional apple, like a rogue baby chimp.

The stubbornness can get me in trouble, but it also helps me achieve things. The other side of the obstinacy coin is tenacity, and I've never needed it more than I do now. In the past it has helped me give up smoking, win awards, demand a good salary, finish novels, and run my business. Of all these things, infertility has by far required the most.

...

I had a dream about being in the audience on an Oprah show last night. She was giving out fertility treatments. There were purple bags under everyone's chairs. She was shouting gleefully at us: 'And you get IVF! And you get IVF! And you get IVF!' and we all went bat-shit crazy.

41

IVF #2

We're going to keep on trucking. Dr G wants us to do another cycle of IVF as soon as possible. It was the most serious I've seen him. He was completely out of character — he didn't even compliment Mike on his sperm.

The good news is that he doesn't think the cyst will be a problem, and he doesn't recommend surgery or bone-crumbling Zoladex. In fact, he said that there is a risk with Zoladex that once you have forced the body into menopause that you can't switch it back on again. That gave me cold chills, like I had only just managed to avoid that happening to me.

What I am not happy with is that he wants to follow the exact same procedure as the last IVF. I argued with him, saying that we surely need to change something if we expect a different result. It's like that crap saying: 'The definition of insanity is trying the same thing over and over again and expecting a different result.' I hate it when people say that. I feel like telling them to read a book. Preferably a dictionary. But I do agree with the sentiment.

Dr G's view is that the cycle went really well. When he said that I think I may have looked at him with my mouth open (unless Mike's elbow in my ribs was meant as congratulations). It's true, said the doc: We made all the numbers and ticked all the boxes. It was a successful cycle, apart from the implantation failure, which is a bit of a gamble on a good day. He thinks we have a good chance in round 2.

Round 2? I thought, as my energy melted onto his tasteful office carpet. Can I honestly put myself through this again? Can we afford it? Can I survive it?

Round 2. I guess I'll put my boxing gloves on. Ding-ding-ding.

...

Walked into VL at 6am for our first scan and bloods for the new IVF cycle and the receptionist asks if it's our first time. I laughed louder than what was appropriate.

The scan was fine and while we were waiting for the blood results we walked up the road to have breakfast. The food was terrible, the coffee was worse. We spoke about death and cancer and not having enough money to realise our dreams of kids and travelling and owning our own time. We walked back to the clinic in that Sandton exhaust fug. Enough bleakness to blot out any ray of morning light, any green of leaf.

It made me think of that time we went for breakfast

at Salvation Café at 44 Stanley after our first AI with the BFG, after a year of trying-not-trying. The food was delicious and we were so optimistic. Our faces were practically bursting with hope. We talked about pregnancy and families, and we brainstormed baby names. I'm sure that when we got up to go the waiters had to hand-vacuum all the glitter we left behind, as if a stripper had exploded at the table.

How times have changed. What is the opposite of glitter? Dust? Ash? It makes sense; the death of a dream.

...

There is a fertility clinic in India that guarantees you a pregnancy or your money back. It is expensive, as you pretty much pay for three IVF cycles upfront, but it's like an insurance policy. You get unlimited treatment until you conceive. I am thinking of moving to India for the foreseeable future. I've always liked saris. And yoga. And butter naan.

...

While I lie pinned to the acupuncturist's table like a life-size voodoo doll, I listen to a fertility meditation to hypnotise my subconscious into falling pregnant. You never know what blockages exist, I read somewhere. I think of it as cleansing my fertility aura. Spiritual detox of the nethers. Just in case. Usually I choose science over silliness, but desperate times, etc. etc. My acupuncturist said it's a good idea. The mind, after all, is a Powerful Thing.

The meditation is lovely to listen to. It's a gentle male voice telling you that you know how to fall pregnant. I love his light Scottish accent, the way he says BEAR-BIE (baby). Think of BAIRDS talking to yer, he says (I do! I always think. I DO hear birds talking to me). Think of yer FEY-verrit food. YOOO ARE GETTING SLEEEEPY.

OUT OF THE IF CLOSET

I believe in sharing my infertility woes with anyone who is willing to listen, and even some who aren't. The more people talk openly about it, the more the subject will be demystified, the less shame there will be for all involved. Infertility shouldn't be taboo. It's a disease, after all. Do people feel ashamed when they are diagnosed with measles? It wasn't your fault you got measles, was it? And it could stop people from giving IFers idiotic advice, like 'just go on a cruise,' or 'avoid caffeine,' because the more of us there are out of the IF closet, the more we can educate people who tell stories of their second-cousin-twice-removed's niece's neighbour's stalker's girlfriend who was told that she'd never be able to fall pregnant but then one day she just 'relaxed' (drank a jug of frozen margarita) and whammo! She was preggers. Isn't it a miracle?!

So I tell pretty much every person I meet about my infertility issues. After all, who doesn't want to hear about devil-uteri and bad eggs?

For example:

Cashier: 'Plestic?'

Me: 'Sorry?'

Cashier: (sighs) 'Plestic beg?'

Me: 'Oh! No thanks. Have a bag here, see? Trying to save the environment, you know.'

Cashier: (yawns, showing a lump of pale pink chewing gum way past its best).

Me: 'For the kids, you know. Do you have kids?' (not waiting for reply) Because I'm trying. We're trying. Been 2 and a half years now. 2 and a half years of treatments. And trying.'

Cashier: 'Shem.'

Me: 'We'll get there, eventually.'

Cashier: (shrugs)

Or

Guy in bar: 'Hey, good-looking. Can I buy you a -'

Me: 'Don't even think about it. I'm married. And even if I wasn't, you'd be wasting your time. I'm a barren wasteland down there. Think Chernobyl. Fukushima. You'd have better luck mating with an Orangutan.'

Guy in bar: 'I was actually speaking to the girl behind you.'

...

The kindness of friends is getting me through this cycle. Last cycle I felt excited, hopeful and poor. Now I'm just poor and getting on with it. Mandie gave me the leather bracelet of hers that I love — it has the outline of a heart stitched into it: a reminder of how far I have come, even if it doesn't always feel like it. I wear it every day, it is my lucky charm. Sitting having my IL IV done, I have a packed breakfast from Mike, a packed lunch from Roela, and quite possibly the best chocolate brownies ever made, from expert baker Avish. Where would I be without this love? I don't want to know the answer.

...

In so much pain I am seeing stars. Shoulder on fire. Insides cramping. Nauseous.

Stimming is not good for me. Counting the days for it to be over.

Have already taken my daily limit of Synap. Only 4pm. I have to take more or I will die. Again, no sleep. Body a wreck. Again, I think which embryo would choose to implant in this hot mess?

...

They say that you should be careful what you wish for. My shoulder was murdering me so I wished that the stimming would be over and now it is. We went for a scan this morning to monitor follicle progress (hoping for 8 — 12, like last time) and to cut a long story short, there was no progress. Two lonely follies floating on the screen. A normal healthy fertile woman would have one follicle without any stimming. I had one, maybe two. After 5 amps of Menopur a day.

It was such a blow. There I am, trucking along with my little purple bag, expecting a normal scan, a normal number of follicles, the go-ahead to keep on going until it's time to trigger, and wham! Knocked sideways by a bad-luck-truck I never saw coming. Serves me right. There was too much unthinking hope in my heart. I should have known. I should have fucking known.

Devastated.

Is that it for us now? Does it mean that my eggs are well and truly finished? *Klaar?* I don't see why else we'd get such a terrible turnout. It's like spending a fortune inviting some friends over to a party that may or may not end in a miracle and they don't bother to come. Except that it's worse, because even bad friends find their way back to you, while my eggs just seem ... well, they just seem finished.

I couldn't handle the news. I started full-out drizzing in Dr G's office. I'm not ready to give up on my (virtually non-existent, as it may seem) fertility. The doc remained calm even while I was doing my worst/best ugly-cry: that hiccupping/hyperventilating weeping that you do (usually in private), nose streaming, mascara doing the Rorschach all over my cheeks. He suggested we see the resident psychologist to work through our disappointment. Too little, too late, I was thinking. A counsellor is not going to be able to un-rotten my eggs.

...

Because I have two good-looking follies (*wolf-whistle*), Dr G doesn't want to 'waste' them. We'll go in for a turkey basting in a few days' time, just in case we get lucky. AIs don't have a high success rate, but it's a better chance than not doing it. We're not hopeful, but what else can we do? Apart from scheduling an appointment to see the psychologist, which I have done. I know that any kind of emotional support has been proven to influence positive outcomes in fertility treatment, so here we come, Crackers Counsellor #2. Here we come, dragging our chronically infertile heels.

THE RIVER

After hours of crying yesterday, I feel sort of cleansed today. I was acting as if the worst had happened and there was nothing we could do, which isn't a true reflection of our circumstances at the moment.

The doc, having inadvertently proven his theory that even if you follow exactly the same process it is possible to get a different result, said that just because my ovaries didn't respond this cycle, it doesn't mean that they won't respond next cycle. This doesn't make any sense to me. I thought that Science Was Science and that Drugs Worked. How are fertility doctors (or any specialists, for that matter) supposed to work in these slippery conditions where 1 + 2 is not always 3? I'm learning that not even science is black and white, and it's frustrating and heartening in equal measures.

So I'm feeling more philosophical about our prognosis. I'm thinking of that school of thought that a man can never step in the same river twice, because the man you are today is not the same as the man you will be tomorrow, and the river, with all its inherent movement, is certainly not the same river, either. If you have constantly changing variables on both sides of the equation, the result may differ from minute to minute. If this is true, and I now I think it is, I may be fertile this very moment. Chances are that I'm not, but now at least the possibility exists.

Dr G wants us to try another round of IVF. Yesterday I was, like, WHY?! It doesn't fucking work! And you call yourself a Man of Science. Don't you know anything? But today I see that there is no other way. Of course we must do another IVF. No matter how rocky the bed, we need to get back into that river.

It is tradition in our house to have a leisurely breakfast on a Sunday morning. First it's tea and rusks, and a reading marathon in bed for me, then up to be barefoot in the kitchen. It's usually a cheese omelette, or poached eggs on sourdough with salsa, rocket and parmesan. Afterwards we have coffee, maybe some chocolate. Sometimes we go for a walk.

Usually it's very pleasant, but sometimes Mike has a bee in his bonnet about something or other, usually to do with the house. Today it was about my business. He started hammering away at me. How much is Pulp earning? Enough to pay all my bills, I said, apart from fertility bills, which we had agreed to take out of the bond once it had demolished our savings. I've always been responsible with money. It's not enough, he said. What am I going to do about it? What are my plans? And variations of these demands, over and over again. I shrug, I'm doing the best I can. My apparent complacency infuriates him.

I know more than anyone that my business has slid this year. It weighs on me every day. That's what happens when you do back-to-back fertility treatments and have your days and energy eaten up by pain. He didn't say anything I hadn't already thought. It's the pressure I put on myself that made me cry, not him, really. And now this conflict between us: this pecking, these splinters. This morning I just feel so hard done by. Infertility has taken so much from me, and without hope of ever getting my baby, it all seems too much of a sacrifice.

Mulligan

Roela came over today and I gossiped shamelessly about Mike and how mean he was to me on the weekend. She said: 'Mike is a WONDERFUL guy, yes?'

'Yes,' I had to say. In general terms, yes. Dammit, yes.

'He has a beautiful soul,' she said. 'Yes?'

'Yes,' I said, begrudgingly. I was sure she was missing the point entirely.

'Now, you love each other very much. You are both under a lot of stress. There are bound to be ructions.'

I wasn't quite sure I knew what 'ructions' were but

it sounded about right, so I nodded.

'So my advice to you then,' she said, 'Is to give him a Mulligan.'

A Mulligan? I searched my mind for the meaning. A cake? A beer? A special kind of blow job?

She explained to me that in golfing, when you are having an otherwise fair game but then you blunder a shot that would ruin your scorecard, your fellow golfers could, if they were in a generous mood, look the other way and let you play the shot again. It could only happen once in a while and should not be turned into a habit. It was against the rules of the game but totally acceptable if you are mates, like Mike and I are.

The concept is good. I'm giving him a Mulligan.

42

FINGERNAILS ON A CHALKBOARD

After a tough few months (years?) I went out last night with Msibi and we blew off some steam. It was a friend's bachelorette. We put on our party dresses, called a taxi, and began drinking. It started off badly: I love women, but I hate all-girl functions. I find that both men and women are better company in each others', well, company. While we were having dinner the girl opposite me was giving me advice on how to fall pregnant, and which dates and positions to make use of if I wanted to gender-pick our baby. I smiled and nodded, not having the energy to engage with her, and more interested in my Mojito than in the mind-numbing conversation. On any other occasion I would have set her straight, but I was there to let my hair down, drink tequila, and dance until the sun came up. Msibi was squeezing my knee under the table but I just patted her hand. It was not something to get upset over, I thought, downing my cocktail. Dinner dragged on like fingernails on a chalkboard with all its grating girly shrieking and fake delight.

211

As soon we were released from the table of torture I beelined to the bar. I needed testosterone and beer and lots of it. Msibi and I danced with each other and whoever else would dance with us. We were flirted with and we flirted back. It was such a release to be (virtually) anonymous, to just be a beergoggle-pretty girl in a short black dress, light years away from endometriosis and depression and infertility. A man bought me a bottle of Moët. I told him that I was happy with the Windhoek Lager I had just ordered, but he insisted. He seemed sexy and funny and charming and if Mike wasn't in my life I probably would have gone home with him. But I am married and I told him so, told him not to waste his champagne or his time on me, that nothing was going to happen; I was the opposite of a sure thing. Not only do I not cheat, I told him, but I don't *want* to cheat. That seemed to make him like me more. I was having a good time flirting. If he wanted to get laid, I said, which I'm sure he did, he'd best move on, and take his champagne with him. He said he'd rather stay and chat to me, and to Msibi, and so we did, sitting, knees touching, laughing for an hour until it was morning and time to go home.

In the taxi home we drove past two roadblocks and high-fived each other for not driving drunk. We passed out in Msibi's bed and woke up hot and hung over. We had borrowed a lot of happiness from the night before, we agreed, looking at each other with our sleep-swollen eyes. I told her what an excellent time I had had. She said: 'You needed to do it.'

Then I remembered the looks from the other girls who had been at the hen party, in the club. Imagined them *skinnering* about how I had reacted to the male attention I had received. *You know she's married,* I can hear them snarling. Their disapproval didn't bother me. Only I knew what my objective had been that night, and I had achieved it without incurring bad karma, and without hurting anyone.

Besides, I've never been into slut-shaming, especially when it comes to my own behaviour. I'm a sexual being and proud of it. One day in high school a friend of a friend told me that someone had said I was a slut. Indignant, I had told my mother. 'Well,' she said, 'Do you sleep with many boys?'

'No!' I said, truthfully. (I was a virgin until I was almost 21. Not due to lack of interest on my side, mind you. I had a high libido and a lot of boyfriends). Even now, at 32, you can count the number of lovers I've had on ... well, two fingers.

'If you're not sleeping around, you're not a slut,' she said, simply. 'They don't know what the word means.'

And now, due to the famous/infamous Slut Walks, the word has lost more of its power. All that said, I'm not looking forward to the pitying glances they are undoubtedly going to be throwing Mike's way at the wedding. Poor man, they'll be whispering, as if he is a cuckold. He doesn't have a clue. And look how nice he is. And stuck with her. That slutty slut-slut.

I told Mike about the man who bought me a bottle of Moët. He said: You must have done something right.

43

Matryoshka

I've been doing some research online about eggs (Yes. My life has become That Sad), and learnt that a female foetus already has her own eggs. Which means that I already existed when my grandmother was pregnant with my mother, in 1950. It's like a Russian Matryoshka doll. Amazing! Also: no wonder I feel so old.

...

So we went for our turkey basting. It was unremarkable in every way. This time, instead of going to a party afterwards, I went straight home and spent the day working in bed. There is absolutely no proof that lying down after AI helps but it felt right.

We went to the fertility psychologist the other day and it was okay. I didn't feel that we got much out of it — after all, it's not like I'm repressing my feelings or not 'processing' my emotions in any way. I talk about it constantly. And when I forget to talk about it for a few days, my shoulder steps in and reminds me. I'm so obsessed with falling pregnant that my emotional processor is in overdrive.

But while I am waiting for said perking up (I'm currently picturing my fallopian tubes like caffeine-baited mongooses) it's best I get on with the doctor's orders and seek professional help of the crackers variety. I think he was more alarmed by my ugly crying jag than he initially let on. I was, like, at least I'm not bottling up my emotions and getting psychosomatic blockage-related illnesses, right? And he was more, like, You Need Help. Full stop. And please clean up that puddle of tears on my office carpet before the next disillusioned couple comes in to write me a cheque.

The counsellor was a lovely, gentle woman. She said one thing that resonated with me. Now that I think about it, perhaps for that it was worth it. She said that even if this AI doesn't work, and even if the third-and-final IVF doesn't work (and that we should obviously be prepared for that outcome — I told her, believe me, I'm prepared. I'm more prepared than a boy scout with OCD) that if we truly want to be parents, it will happen. She wasn't talking about airy-fairy 'just think positive' but rather, if you are committed enough to the outcome, it will happen. There are many ways to become parents. I'll say that again, because it is important: There are many ways to become parents. Our first choice (natural conception) didn't work, and we are entitled to our grief over that. We didn't want to do fertility treatments, but when it came down to having treatments or not having children, treatments suddenly became an option. In the same way, if the treatments don't work (and it looks as though we are heading in that direction), we can adopt. It may not be our first choice, but when everything else is exhausted, it will become a good option. It has been a wonderful choice of action for millions of people all over the world: (Yes, Brangelina, I'm talking about you.)

She wasn't saying, like Fertile Myrtles the world over seem to love to spout: '*Ag* man, just adopt!'

It was a more considered version. She was saying, adoption may become the answer for you. And if that time comes, you will be happy to have that option.

In other words, whatever happens, if we are totally committed to becoming parents, we will become parents. There is a beauty and simplicity in that thought that I really liked. Not that it's not difficult to take on board — that I may never be pregnant, give birth, breastfeed, have our own biological children — it's still heartbreaking to me. But. But. But. There are always options. There is no end of the road in sight, and that is a consolation.

44

RAVENCLAWS

Another thing the counsellor said is that the grief pattern observed in couples grappling with infertility is similar to Post Traumatic Stress Disorder. While that sounds a bit hammed-up, I did take her point. PTSD is a haunting kind of anxiety: a lighter-than-air grey-coloured raven that sits on your shoulder. He's hardly noticeable until there is some kind of trigger, and then he sinks his talons into you. You do what you can to get rid of him, to coax him away, but he persists. Most dreadfully: his poisonous talons persist.

Normal grief, like you would experience after losing someone, usually follows a linear process. But in the midst of trying to conceive while infertile, you're not allowed the chance to heal and move on. Instead, you have ravenclaws: you're stuck in a grief cycle like a hamster on a wheel, like the spinning beachball of death, with no end in sight, and this can become overwhelming.

She added that my physical pain, in conjunction with my psychic pain, makes it worse. Like an endless loop-de-loop of anticipating pain and experiencing pain, and no downtime to recover. Psychologically speaking, she said, it's asking for trouble.

I appreciated her acknowledging my pain. It seems stupid that I should require this. I didn't know I did, but it made me feel better; less lonely. The pain is alienating. No one I know has chronic pain, and when I talk about it to people I can feel that they don't understand it (why would they?). Even though there was nothing she could do about it, I feel like she 'got it'.

Sometimes my more paranoid side wonders if people think I am imagining the pain — or worse, making it up — in order to express the psychological pain of infertility. I hate this idea. It shouldn't bother me, but it does. It's, like, not only has the universe punched me in the face, but people think I am crying because it hurt my feelings, instead of because I have a broken nose and it's stinging like hell. Yes, my feelings are hurt, and that's not easy, either, but please don't undermine my punched-up face, especially when I have another fist coming next month, and the next month, and the month after that.

I try everything to get my raven to let go. I throw prayers and promises like scraps of carrion in the air for him, but he knows my tricks better than I know them myself, and his ghost-like barbs never leave my shoulder.

...

Mike and I feel like we shouldn't bankrupt our

future for another round of IVF. But in the end it's all just talk. Of course we'll do another round. One last round. We can't afford not to. We'll borrow the money from our much-abused bond. It's already a 30-year loan (it was the only way we could afford the house) and it doesn't look like it will be paid off any time soon. What's 30 years between friends?

In my email update to the Mike Junior fans I asked everyone to buy lottery tickets.

Msibi wrote back: 'Absolutely! R30 million next weekend.'

Me: 'Think of all the babies I can have for R30 mill!'

Msibi: 'Ha ha! Lotto Lawrence.'

Me: 'One day is one day.'

CHUNK OF CHANGE

My mom gave me a large chunk of change to help with treatment costs. I am so grateful. Her timing is perfect — I'm going for the pregnancy test in a few days' time so the money will act as a bit of a financial (and emotional) cushion in the event of a negative result. A Big Fat Negative will still hurt, but it will hurt less. I feel as if a weight has been lifted from my shoulders.

The gift is made all the more poignant through knowing that my mom doesn't have a lot of cash to throw around. She has been a teacher all her adult life, and a single mother since Denton and I were smallies. She has done so much for us, sacrificed so much for us, and her generosity inspires me. I want to tell her to keep the money, but I won't, because A) she won't take it back, she is as stubborn as I am, and B) I am, quite simply, desperate for it.

Knowing how hard she works for her money and thinking of her generosity makes me feel emotional. What a gift it will be if it helps me conceive. What a travesty if it is wasted.

. . .

Seen today:

"Life is short. Smile while you still have teeth."

. . .

Slightly more nervous than excited for the pregnancy test tomorrow. I have no symptoms of either pregnancy or period, so in theory it could go either way. I realise the chances of success are slight, but there is always a small voice at the back of my mind, a cheerleader with pom-poms, that says 'This may be the month.'

When I shrug her off she shouts: 'Give me a B! Give me an F! Give me a BFP!'

45

Knock Down Some Walls

Our blood test today was negative. We don't want to lose hope, but it feels like we are swimming against the tide.

We have plans outside of getting pregnant (I know, you'd never guess!), like more travelling, and renovating the house, which we have placed on hold for almost two years. We needed the money for the treatments. I haven't been to the optometrist/dentist/dermatologist for the same amount of time, not wanting to spend a cent of our medical savings account on anything but getting pregnant. My glasses are nine years old and it goes without saying that they don't work as well as they used to, but who cares about a pair of glasses when your biggest dream is hanging in the balance? Who needs to read sub-titles, anyway?

But we are beginning to feel hemmed in by these un-realised goals, and after the Big Fat Negative today we both felt like saying a big 'Fuck You' to reality at large. If we by chance had a big neon sign — Las Vegas style, with blinking lights — of an erect middle finger in-between an 'F' and a 'U', we'd put it up outside our house and switch it on.

So in that vein, we are thinking, fuck it, let's just do it anyway. We are throwing caution to the wind and taking all the cash we have in our access bond and renovating the house. We need to change the energy in this house, smash some windows, knock down some walls. I know that building and renovating can be really stressful, but I'm feeling, pssh! Infertility is stressful. Spending your life's savings on treatments that don't work is stressful. I'm ready for a new type of stress.

It will be good to have a project we can work on together. Something (else) to talk about.

. . .

I got a huge book order for Pulp today. Felt like dropping to my knees and thanking whichever god was listening. I really needed some good news and seeing a big fat wad of money like that coming in does wonders for your spirit.

. . .

Chris has also given us some money towards our final IVF. It was so generous of him, it touched me deeply, I couldn't help but give him a big hug, despite him not being a hugger.

46

THE PLOT THICKENS

So here we are so far with this plot:

The Plot (WIP)

1. Wedding! Honeymoon! Off the pill! So excited! Life is Awesome!

...

22. Begin 2nd of 3 medicated cycles. Get faux morning sickness. Awesome. BFN.

23. Have 3rd of 3 medicated cycles. Get extremely sick. Period is late. BFN.

24. Start first IVF! Eeeeeek! Exciting! Stimming works! Fertilisation works! Transfer works! Implantations fails. BFN.

25. Get 2nd opinion from Clinic B. Don't like 2nd opinion. Go back to VL.

26. Start 2nd round of IVF. Stimming is a bust. Labelled a 'poor responder'. IVF converted to IUI. BFN.

27. Out of money, out of hope.

28. Get a bit of money, get a bit of hope.

28. Decide to do one last round of IVF. 3rd time lucky?

The first chapter in 'The Memory of Water' is a boy recounting the morning his sister drowned while they were swimming in a nearby river. Water and drowning remain a theme throughout the book, as the protagonist's life spirals out of control.

A few months ago, while I was trying to come up with the title, I thought about Stevie Smith's poem, 'Not Waving But Drowning'. It's flawless. It's about someone who is drowning, motioning for help, but bystanders think he is just playing around and ignore his flailing, and he drowns. The poem is poignant perfection. How many people feel that way, I think, as they flail?

Drowning is so often used as metaphor in writing. A short story I read this week that describes a young woman as being pulled under, the evening sky like 'pink water'. I thought, yes, while reading it, I know that pink water. I swim in that pink water. Sometimes I go under, too.

When we were around 16, Pin and I went swimming in the sea at Gonubie beach, in East London. It was something I had done hundreds of times before. Gonubie had been our family's December holiday spot since before I was born. The water is cold there, and there are sharks, but on that particular day everything seemed so warm and wonderful, the water so calm, that we spent ages floating around far out, past the splashing suncream-covered children and the muddy dunkers and the bodysurfers and the underwater couples stealing furtive caresses of each other's cold, tight skin. We were buoyed by our good moods, being in the middle of a holiday of boys and beer and freedom after a year of being stifled by a conservative boarding school.

An undercurrent was sweeping us further and further out. I lost sight of Pin, but I didn't worry. I started swimming slowly back to shore, or rather, I went through the motions of swimming but I stayed in the same place. Before I had time to worry, a lifeguard in a kayak popped up, as if by magic, to rescue me. I don't need rescuing, I laughed, I'm not in trouble. I'm a strong swimmer. Unbeknownst to me, people had started gathering on the beach to watch the drama unfold, including a puzzled Pin who had been at my side just moments before. He showed me where to climb out, at the rocks, so that I wouldn't have to fight against the sea. When I was safely out of the water, I thanked him off-handedly, as if I were in fact the one doing him a favour, and attempted to walk away gracefully, proceeding to cut my foot on a rock. If only the poor protagonist in Stevie Smith's poem had such an insistent lifesaver on duty, he may still be alive.

. . .

My absolutely beautiful nephew, Denton's son, was born today. We all rushed through to the hospital in Pretoria together to meet him. It was so strange in so many ways. It was a planned C-section, yet Denton wasn't there for the birth. I can't imagine that.

K was glowing; baby Cam was, I think, the sweetest newborn I have ever seen, apart from Pin's Ben. My mom got to meet her first and only grandchild.

My God, it was difficult for me. I kept wondering if a giant crack was going to appear in the earth's surface to swallow me up, or a sudden storm would come along and electrocute me. Being in the moment was so painful. The unspoken apology on my brother's face, the pity on my mother's. I wanted to tell them that this day wasn't about me, but, of course, they knew that. That is what made it so sad.

It was so difficult until I finally held him — and then all the resentment melted away. He was perfect. Absolutely perfect, and I loved him immediately. It was the first time I understood how love could be transformative. In a short, precious moment the bittersweetness of the day lost its bite.

Mike looked so lovely holding him, so strong and gentle, that I wanted to cry. Perhaps I did, a little. It was just so poignant a picture. My mom moved closer to me; a show of compassion.

In the car on the way back to Jo'burg D's new

girlfriend sighed dramatically and said: 'That was SUCH a difficult day for me.' And I thought: Chick, you haven't got a clue. I kept quiet and looked out of the window. Mike squeezed my hand.

LITTER

Our looming anniversary is making me remember how we got engaged. It's a funny/awkward story.

Not being a big fan of marriage, for the following reasons: (Yay! Lists!)

1. I don't believe that humans were meant to be monogamous over the long term.

2. I believe that you are a vastly different person at 20 than you are at 30 and 40 and 50. You may want to link arms in sickness and in health now, but you will be two very different people soon. Who knows if you will even get on in 10 years time, never mind want to shag each other, or look at each other over scrambled eggs at the breakfast table.

3. I think it's seriously old-fashioned.

4. I think that (like religion) people do it unthinkingly, because their parents did it. I think people get married without really considering what they are doing and why — they are obediently following the ABC of being a 'grown-up'. It's even worse when people have children for this reason.

5. I think it can be the death-knell for many relationships as people stop trying; like the marriage contract is a licence for taking your partner for granted.

6. I want to be with Mike because I want to be with Mike, not because we are legally bound or owe it to each other to 'make it work'. Plus, divorce is like a Louis Vuitton tote: ugly, expensive, and full of baggage.

7. I see broken marriages everywhere I look, like the ruins of some sad romantic town. My parents (twice for my dad), Mike's parents, family friends, aunts and uncles, etc. etc. If they couldn't keep it together, then how will we?

8. I believe in the Zen way of looking at relationships: that they are good for as long as they are good, and then they are over. So simple and elegant in its truth.

9. I question the very act of a person asking the other person to sign a piece of paper to legally bind them. The idea is nothing short of bizarre. Why would you do that? What are you scared of? What is next — asking your dog to sign a contract that he will be your best friend until death do you part?

10. I'm a feminist and marriage has not been kind to our cause. It's a man-made institution that is mostly patriarchal and pro-male, designed, I believe, to keep wild, juicy women safely at home, treating stains, darning socks and trying new 'exciting' recipes.

Mandie and Avish agree with me on the whole, (they've been together since the dawn of days but there are no wedding bells in their immediate future), although they have their own reasoning, but Mike was on the fence. He is a feminist, too, whether he wants to admit it or not (I wouldn't be with someone who isn't a feminist), so he understands, but the caveman/romantic in him wanted to do it, anyway. After many colourful debates among the four of us, I thought that the matter had been put to (its non-matrimonial) bed.

One of my favourite quotes comes from a story that Chris tells. He says a friend of his, at a party, once said: "I'd hate to be unhappily married. I'm happily married and it's shit."

Scene change! Mike and I are walking on a white beach of paradise, awe-inducing cliffs that jut magnificently out of the serene sea. We're in Thailand, on a remote island. It's early morning. We're taking photographs while we're the only ones on the beach. Mike grabs my arm, tells me to look down. He nudges a piece of litter with his foot.

'What's that?' he asks. The hot glare from the white sand hurts my eyes.

'Leave it,' I say, 'it's litter or … something.' It was odd, like a small white rock. I wanted to keep walking, keep shooting, but he held me back with a gentle hand. He picked up the object, which I now saw was a piece of paper around a stone. He unwrapped it in front of my eyes, like a gift, or a treasure map. When I saw it was his handwriting inside I was confused. How the — ? What the — ? And then I saw it was a love letter from him to me and when I looked up from reading it he was kneeling in front of me with a diamond ring, and he asked me to marry him.

I think everyone on the island must have stopped what they were doing — chopping down coconuts, repairing their tuk-tuks, pulling on their slops — and wondered what that strange sound was (it was my mind being blown). I didn't speak for a while. I was probably as pale as the beach sand we were standing on. I probably turned invisible, like those jellyfish that change colour according to their surroundings. Poor Mike. Can you imagine you ask someone to marry you and POOF! they disappear, right in front of your eyes.

Turned out he had to ask me a few times before he got a comprehensible answer. I said yes. We crossed paths with another couple a few moments later and they yelled: 'Congratulations!' and I thought, Oh Holy Moses, what have I done? I was quiet for the rest of the day, staring at the excessively cheerful glinting diamond on my finger, waiting for my mind to un-boggle.

I joke with Mike that the reason I agreed to marry him was the size of the diamond. It's a *grappie*, but there is truth in it. What kind of person, who is usually careful with money, spends a truckload of cash on having a ring made for a person he pretty much knows is going to turn him down? I like that person. That person has resolve (and balls). In fact, I like that person so much I married him. If the diamond had been half the size? Who knows.

That would have been a *kak* holiday.

ANNIVERSARY

After a difficult day yesterday it's our second wedding anniversary today (eight years together) and Mike wrote a letter to me in our anniversary book. He said that we will get through this and we'll have our baby. Despite a few (expected) rough patches this fuck-circus has been good for us. You know when they say bad things are good for building your character? This nightmare has built character for this particular tag-team. I know a lot of relationships don't survive infertility, but it has brought us closer. I'm lucky to have him, even if he is a teetotalling pescatarian.

He wrote that we'll do this thing, and that I must keep writing 'Mike Jnr' in the sand.

...

We flew down to Port Elizabeth for Jack's funeral. Of course Rosemary (his widow of more than 30 years) is terribly sad, but the rest of the family don't seem too upset. He had a fantastic innings at 91, a wonderful, full life, and after the stroke put him in a wheelchair a year or so ago, he told us that he was ready to move on.

It was what I think everyone wishes their funeral could be: a warm-hearted celebration instead of a wail-fest followed by a terribly boring tea party.

While remembering the good times, and the jokes, there is always someone who takes it too far. This someone is usually Mike's middle brother Simon, but today it was Chris. Jack had been a sanitary inspector all his working life, and at lunch Chris asked his widow what she would be doing with the ashes. 'Scatter them on the tip, will you, Rose?'

Thank goodness she is deaf in one ear.

I did end up crying at the funeral. Chris delivered a funny and warm eulogy listing all Jack's achievements, including three wives and five children. When it was the priest's turn to speak about Jack, he said that he had been blessed with so many children because he had been 'good at it.'

The pre-infertile me would have sniggered. Good at what? I would whisper to Mike, elbowing him in the ribs. Shagging? Catholicism? Good at not watching TV? More like: bad at contraception.

But the infertile me knew what the priest meant. He had meant that God blessed Jack with so many children because he was a good man, and I took exception to that. To be fair, I take exception to most of what comes out of religious people's mouths (except for that love-your-neighbour stuff, although I don't find a lot of them preach or practice this). So if I were to extrapolate his idea, he would be saying that I am not blessed with kids because I am not good, or not good enough? I wish I could say that I felt the invigorating spark of righteous anger, that I took the man aside and gave him a talking-to, a real what-for, but his words saddened me. Seemed to drain the life out of me. I felt cold and empty, as though my back and hip bones had been replaced with chilled metal while I wasn't looking. In the depressing church hall afterwards, the rain spitting on the roof, no amount of tepid tea or cardboard sandwiches could fill me up.

— Note to priest: Don't take it too personally. Have you heard the joke: Q: How do you offend an Infertile? A: Open your mouth.

(Granted, it's not the funniest joke, but I'm trying, for a change, to be gracious.)

— Note to self: Never attend another religious ceremony without a topped-up hip flask.

...

Back in Jo'burg today, we visited baby Cam. So wonderful/joyful/difficult to hold him and feel that bond of blood. So close, but not close enough. He looks like an adorable elf in his little blue hat, and has Denton's big ears. Pathetically, I didn't want to let him go.

NOTHING MATTERS

I'd like to add a few more questions to the Google screening for depression.

10. Do you sometimes feel like a walking zombie?

11. Do you find it difficult to get up in the morning?

12. Are you loathe to leave the house?

13. Do you often just think 'Fuck It'?

14. Have you turned into a sullen shell of a person?

15. Do you often find yourself in an existential crisis, thinking 'what is the point of anything', and not finding a satisfactory answer?

16. Does the world look grey?

17. Do you have these words stamped on your forehead?: 'NOTHING MATTERS'

...

Driven to distraction by my last cycle, I went back to my GP. I needed fresh eyes on my pain. Also, I needed a new script for my favourite painkillers.

My stash of Synap F is coming to an end and I get a panicky feeling when I see the tablets disappearing. I start off with a big white box of them. I think I have plenty but then on a rough night I'll count them and can't imagine where they have gone. It's as though I have elves visiting in the middle of the night but instead of doing the dishes / sorting my underwear / cleaning the oven they plunder my pills instead. Little hopped-up bastards.

I told the doc I'm desperate (again). I couldn't sleep at all last night. The hours and hours of empty night-time are doing my head in. He wrote me a new prescription and referred me to a pain specialist.

A pain specialist? Music to my ears. What fresh, minty, glittering magic is this? I never knew such a thing existed. She is clearly very good at her job because just phoning for an appointment made me feel better. Or maybe that was the newly acquired box of Synap Forté I had in my paws.

47

Dr Finegan & the Pain Drawer

Are your eyes watering? Do you feel like there is too much light in the room? That's because Dr Finegan, Pain Specialist Esquire, has arrived in all her gleaming glory. Sunshine is beaming out of her every orifice. She has rainbows emanating from her (otherwise ordinary) face. Sparkling ink from her sparkling pen sparkles on her sparkling prescription pad. This is how I remember her in retrospect. In real life, it went more like this:

Finegan: 'How much pain are in you in, on a scale of 1 − 10?'

Me: (eyes dulled by pain and general life-jaded-ness) 'Depends on the time of the month.'

Finegan: 'How bad can it get?'

Me: '7? 8? 9? Five hundred and eleventy?'

Finegan: 'Does it make you feel suicidal?'

Me: 'Not today.'

Finegan: 'On a bad day?'

Me: 'Not suicidal, but ...'

Finegan: 'Like you don't want to live anymore?'

Me: 'Like I can't live with it anymore.'

Finegan: 'Depressed?'

Me: 'I wouldn't say 'depressed' depressed. But maybe a little. Okay, I probably am, a bit.'

Finegan: 'Chronic pain and depression go hand-in-hand. It's a chemical thing. When we treat your pain you'll feel better all round.'

(She made it seem so simple, like eating a sandwich when you're hungry. You don't need to question the hunger, wonder why you are so hungry, beat yourself up for being hungry, ask why the universe made you so damn hungry. Take a Google test to make sure that you are, in fact, hungry. All you need to do is eat the sandwich.)

Finegan: 'What are you on at the moment?'

Me: 'I was on Myprodol but it burnt a hole in my stomach.'

Finegan: 'Pssh! Myprodol is for amateurs.'

Me: 'I'm on Synap Forté now and it works a lot better. But lately I can't stay on top of the pain anymore without overdosing.'

Finegan: 'Good. Synap is good. But you need NSAIDS.'

Me: 'En-what-what?'

Finegan: 'Non Steroidal Anti Inflammatories. They're the bomb. (Okay she didn't really say 'the bomb'). Endometriosis is an inflammatory condition. You need to douse the flame before it becomes a raging fire.'

Me: (nods head, starting to feel a little bit in love with the exceptionally wise lady sitting on the other side of the desk.)

Finegan: 'We just have to be careful of not interfering with your ovulation.'

Me: (She cares about my ovulation. Cartoon hearts shoot out of my eyes.)

She wrote out three pages of prescriptions and two A4 pages of instructions. How to take the pills, when, how to combine them.

Me: 'It's referred pain. Does that make it harder to treat?'

Finegan: 'Not really. Here, take this stack of papers to the pharmacy and get your dope on.'

Me: 'Wow. That's a serious amount of schedule 6 drugs.'

Finegan: 'Let me be clear. Our objective is to get you pain-free. Not to manage your pain. To get you pain-free.'

Me: (starts crying)

It seemed impossible, until now. How I love Dr Finegan. You know that battleground medic with the morphine injection pen I fantasise about? I had just met him. He turned out to be a middle-aged woman in a cream blouse. With rainbows coming out of her face.

C'est La Vie, Nipplecaps

I got all my new painkillers (and a few suspicious looks) from the pharmacy up the road. I think they might have actually called Finegan's office to make sure the script was legit. I opened my eyes wide and smiled my best non-junkie smile, showing teeth and everything. The pharmacist took a step back, as if I might bite him.

When I arrived home with my bounty, I sat on the bed and got to know the different pills. I studied Finegan's strategy. I feel hopeful. I think that this is going to work. Mike got home to see me surrounded by hundreds of pills. A kid in a candy store.

I needed to make space for the candy in my bedside table drawer. Out went the Myprodol, the chinese meds, the hand cream. There was still not enough space, so I had to move (ahem) some other stuff, too. It used to be my sex drawer — now, it's my pain drawer. *C'est la vie*, nipplecaps. You've been replaced, for now. Don't take it too personally. We'll always have Paris. Or whatever. Pass the pills.

READ THE FUCKING MAIL

After every important development (or as I like to call it, 'Plot Twist!') I send an email to the Mike Jnr Fan Club appraising them of the farce my life has become. Apart from the support I get in response, which can't be underestimated, it also means that I don't have to repeat my sob story again and again. I have become so brittle that I roll my eyes at anyone who asks if there is news. 'Don't you read the emails?' I want to demand. I have gone from wanting to speak about only my fertility issues to not wanting to talk about them at all. It's boring as shit. I'm so over it. News? There's nothing new, or you'd know about it. You want an update? Read the fucking mail.

I get it, okay? I get that they want to talk about it. An email isn't enough. Besides, they don't understand the terms I use. They want to get a feeling of how we are coping. It's easy to put on a brave face and press 'send', and quite another having the actual conversation. They want to probe the possibilities, they want to know what the real story is. But I'm not up to it anymore. I'm not up to making other people feel better about our situation. I'm not up to hearing any more fertility advice from people who don't have a cooking clue. Think of it this way: by not talking about it over a nice dinner, you will not inadvertently say something stupid, and I will not inadvertently stab you with the butter knife. You're welcome.

All I want to do is be on my own, reading, or writing, or destroying what is left of my brain with TV. If I absolutely have to see people, I want to drink. I want to drink enough to put some distance between myself and this tedium I can't seem to escape.

I've just read over what I've written. I used to be easy-going, gracious, despite my hang-ups; (sometimes too) quick to laugh. Who is this person? This sad, bitter bitch.

48

BLUE HAZE, OR, UNHAPPY PILLS

I started Trepiline two days ago. It's an interesting drug because it was first manufactured as an anti-depressant, but was found to have excellent analgesic and sleep-inducing properties. It's not sold as a happy pill anymore (there are far more sophisticated ones out there now) and I can see why. When Dr Finegan told me about it I thought, Awesome, I could do with some happy pills. Turns out they should be called UNhappy pills.

It's chronic medication, so you have to start taking it gradually, a quarter of a tiny blue pill every night, whether you are in pain or not, and when you feel like you have adjusted to it, you up your dose. I looked at the speck of blue in my palm, dubious. How was this grain of powder going to do anything?

On the first night I took it at 10pm and BAM! Slept for nine solid hours. It was beautiful, apart from the hangover, which lasts the whole day. I'm still living in the blue haze. It's like being darted. I would seriously recommend it to anyone who has problems sleeping, unless they actually need to function the next day.

I catch myself sitting in front of my laptop, tea long cold, staring vacantly at my screen, as if someone has eaten my brain. Working is difficult, reading, too. Writing is impossible. I can't hold a thought in my head for long enough to write it down. My appetite (for anything) is gone. Only one thing is clear: I wasn't depressed before. I wasn't close to depressed. I was just sad. This blue haze, THIS is what depression feels like. No energy, no joy, no hope. I know it's only temporary, until I get used to the drug, but that doesn't stop the overwhelming feeling of bleakness I feel. Before, on a bad day, I didn't *want* to get out of bed in the morning. Now, I feel like I *can't* get out of bed. It takes every ounce of willpower I possess to drag myself up and into the shower. Washing my hair is out of the question. There's no way I have the energy to lift my arms for that long.

FRACTURED

Sitting in the garden this morning, trying to explain this utter despair to Mike. I've never been good at expressing my feelings verbally. It's even harder when you have dark cobwebs embroidering your brain.

I can't get on top of the pain today. I've taken everything I'm allowed but still my ribcage feels fractured. Thoughts are fractured, too. This life is like a stuttering home video with the sound turned low. There is nothing to be done except wait for this terrible Trepiline to start working.

Mike says I need to go out, see people. It will make me feel better. Have a drink; a conversation. Take my mind off it. Sometimes that used to work; it used to distract me from the pain. But this is different. I told him I'm not even up to stepping out the front door, never mind 'going out'. All I want to do is hug my knees, as if to catch my breath. I want to stare at the television so that I don't have to think. I want to sleep until this nightmare is over.

He doesn't understand the depth of this darkness. How could he? He said: Your friends will stop asking. You'll lose them. I barked a bitter laugh. I said: Don't you see? I don't care. About anything. I am the breaker of my own heart.

...

This is why I need to stay alive:

1. All the books I have yet to read, all the movies I have yet to see.

2. Friends and family, although I'm hardly adding much value to their lives at the moment.

3. I can't imagine that this is the last chocolate bar I will ever eat. If I stay alive I will get to eat more. Ditto for great food, wine, etc.

4. I want to see what my garden looks like this summer.

5. I want to be around when my first book is published.

6. All the stories and books I have yet to write.

7. My bucket list (mostly travel-related: the countries I have yet to see).

8. My fuck-it list.

9. The chance, no matter how small, that I will one day be pain-free.

10. The chance, no matter how small, that I will one day have a child.

...

Once, in Zanzibar, I stood on a massive urchin while swimming. The spines stuck right into my sole, their spikes buried in my flesh. I had to crawl out of the sea on all fours. Mike and Avish carried me to a nearby beach bar and I sat drinking a beer in my bikini while they plied the long black quills out, leaving the barbs under my skin. For the rest of the holiday I felt those spurs in my heel with every step, like walking on nails. How misleading the vision of that sparkling warm ocean was: how warm and welcoming.

LITTLE BLACK BOOK

Dr Finegan suggested I keep a 'pain diary' to monitor our progress and to make it easier to figure out which drugs are working for me. Also, to keep from overdosing. So in addition to this journal, I now have a little black book in my pain drawer, which I have to fill out when I take something. It doesn't make for pleasant reading.

The Hours Clock By

Dare I say it? I'm feeling better today. The pain is still humming in the background of everything I do, but the blue haze has lifted. I can think. I can concentrate for long enough to get a few things done. Best of all, I seem to have some energy. I spent the morning gardening: lots of hard pruning and cutting away dead parts. Then a bit of tidying up and planting slips and other things. Watering. I am buoyed by the continuing cycle of nature — it is heartening. Hopeful. Life goes on, even in the bleakest time, the hours clock by, the blossoms burst, the annuals go to seed.

I had the most delicious beer afterwards, sitting in the middle of the garden in my old bikini top and my muddied shorts, sand under my nails. Felt almost like myself again. It was good.

I think I'll try to write a bit tonight. I want to take advantage of the energy, the clarity. My new novel lies neglected, untouched for weeks. It is at risk of falling away.

49

GIVING UP THE GHOST

One of my favourite authors, Hilary Mantel, wrote a memoir called 'Giving Up the Ghost,' about her devastating endometriosis and infertility. Although I ordered it the moment I heard about it, it stayed at the bottom of my reading pile. I had not felt strong enough to read it, but now I'm sorry that I didn't read it sooner.

I don't use the word 'devastating' lightly. It not only ravaged her insides, but her fertility and spirit, too. When I read about her symptoms, her terrible thoracic pain, I knew it was diaphragmatic endometriosis. She was describing my pain, but worse, because it was in a time before she could find a Googlenosis, or a doctor skilled enough to find the problem. Instead, the bizarreness of the condition confounded her, and confounded her doctors, and when no (apparent) physical problem was found, they guessed it had to be psychological, and put her on psychoactive drugs that almost ruined her mind altogether. Eventually, at 27, they would botch a surgery on her: there was the deceitful promise of no more pain, but also 'no children'. She was at such a tender age so mishandled and so patronised, she was at risk of losing everything. She says that they 'confiscated' her fertility. I imagine her, waif-like, lying in that cool white hospital bed, bleeding, bereft. The ghost would have to be put to bed: there would be no Catriona (the name she had picked for the daughter she would never have), there wouldn't even be the leisure to decide if she wanted babies or not. There would just be what was: her traitorous body, her insides sliced over and over again by the intractable pain.

Despite her tragedy she writes with such candour and such incisive wit. I was weeping for her, laughing with her, knocked by her prose at every turn. The poetry of heartbreak. At night, now, I check under my (metaphysical) bed. I grapple in the dark, searching for my own ghosts. The book has rattled my soul.

...

I have a wonderful massage therapist/reflexologist. We use to work together at The Jupiter Drawing Room when I was still a whippersnapper of an art director and she was an account manager. We have since both left advertising and found our respective grooves. H's hands are The Best. The fact that she's a lovely person is a bonus. She soothes me with her kind words and spends extra time massaging the babymaker part of my feet.

As you can probably guess, after two years of treatment, my ankles are in peak condition.

MY TRIBE

We're down at San Lameer.

Mothers' Day was horrible. After years of trying to conceive, a friend on the support forum miscarried that morning. On Mothers' Day. I used so see such wonder in the world. Where has it gone?

It's my birthday so I'm trying to Cheer The Fuck Up. Mike planned a special day for me, a whole itinerary starting with a picnic on the beach — salmon and croissants — and ending with a hot stone massage. Later we're going for dinner at Trattoria La Terazza. He is being so lovely.

This holiday I've been trying to get into it, trying to enjoy the time away, but really, mostly, I've been plastering a smile on my face and going through the motions. Trying not to feel sorry for myself. Trying to act as if I am okay. It's for everyone's benefit.

The only place I can really be honest about everything is here and on the forum. No one understands infertility like a fellow infertile. You don't have to worry about anyone thinking you are selfish, or obsessed, or feeling sorry for yourself. They are always there for you, no matter what. They are indispensable. They are my tribe.

. . .

I babysat my nephew tonight. K had a work function and I told her before he was born that she should consider me permanently on call. He is the sweetest baby. I cuddled him for ages, fed him, and put him down to sleep without a whimper (from him). I had a large glass of wine. I was whimpering plenty.

Penis Day in Japan

Mandie sent me an email today about the *Hōnen Matsuri* festival in Japan, AKA Penis Day (I know what you're thinking — is it Big In Japan?). Celebrated every March 15th in Komaki, the townsfolk haul out a large wooden phallus to give three cheers to fertility and renewal. They reckon it's why they have consistently good harvests and a bounty of babies. I think it's only right that I make a pilgrimage. There is all-you-can-drink *sake* and a 2.5m, 250kg (it must be said, artfully sculpted) giant wooden penis. Plus you get to throw some rice-cakes around. What is not to love? Bananas (all shapes and sizes) covered in chocolate and sprinkles! Dicks-on-sticks! Pigs in blankets! Penis-shaped buddhas! Why is it the first time I have heard of this?!

50

JUNKIE

Today has been the lowest point so far in my life. You know when you hear addicts' stories about how they hit rock-bottom before they made a change in their lives? Well, that's me. My psyche is a downtrodden junkie lying in a gutter that smells of piss and vomit, surrounded by dirty needles and used pregnancy test sticks. It has track marks all the way up its arm (Menopur? Cetrotide? Ovidrel?) and an empty wallet. No, not an empty wallet, but an empty pocket where the wallet used to be, because it sold its wallet for one last fix. One last gamble, one roll of the dice. Look at the bruises all over its body, look at its hair falling out. Why is the skin so bad? It is like the 'AFTER' picture in a poster advertising the ill effects of abusing crystal meth, or heroin addiction. There should be these posters warning about infertility, too. Before and After. Like 'Happily Ever After', but the reverse. Rewind the fairy tale, and the princess gets turned into a slave. My psyche lies there, motionless, its chest hardly rising with breath. A passerby kicks it, and still it does not move.

...

I had a mini-breakdown yesterday, as you could probably tell. There are good days and bad days in the fuck-circus my life has become, and yesterday was the worst day so far. My shoulder was sore, and I didn't feel like dealing with it. I took my laptop into the lounge and tried to work there, in front of the TV, to distract myself. Painkillers, hot water bottle, tea, TV, and a promise to myself not to give in to it, not to cry. I had work to do. Money to earn, a life to live.

So what if I'm infertile? I asked myself. It's not the end of the world, even if it feels like it is. Maybe I'll never be pregnant. Maybe I'll never be a mother. Maybe I don't deserve to be a mother. If this is the worst thing that has ever happened to me then I should probably count myself 'lucky.' There are people all over the world in more pain than I am. Enough with the all-consuming self-absorbed self-pitying drama. I am sick to death of it. Pathetic.

Oprah came on, and I was half-watching it in the background of my work, until this story came on about this little boy who was abused by his parents. They would lock him in a cupboard for hours on end, sometimes overnight. There would be fencing wire around him, and a dog chain, so that he couldn't sit down. He would get so tired that he would fall asleep and the wire would cut into his underarms and throat. They would starve him. Sometimes his step-sister was able to smuggle Cheerios in.

He was 6 years old when they found him and helped him. Six. That's still a baby. He trusted his parents, he didn't know any better. His biological mother abandoned him to chase drugs. She was fertile. I'm not. At first I cried for the boy. I cried and cried. Those trusting eyes. Heartbreaking. I thought: no more treatments, we must adopt. Then, later, I cried for myself. What kind of world are we living in that that family was given a child while I sit here, with wide open arms and an empty uterus? I have so much love to give. How can you believe in a god that orchestrates life so very badly? It's not about you, a voice remonstrates. It's my life, I shout back. It fucking well is about me.

51

What Infertility Has Given Me

What infertility has taken away:

1. My trust in the universe: the belief that there actually is someone running this freak show, including:

2. My belief in karma, or rather, that good things happen to good people, and vice versa, and

3. My belief that if you work hard enough to attain a goal you will get it.

4. My ability to go a day without either experiencing or anticipating pain.

5. My appearance: hormonal break-outs, handfuls of hair loss, fever blisters, wrinkles. Sometimes I look at my reflection and wonder how I have aged so quickly in the last two years. I look and feel a decade older than I am.

6. On a bad day: energy to work, to write, to love.

7. My hard-earned money: lots and lots of savings. The assurance of having money in the bank.

8. Time! Time spent in waiting rooms, having scans, waiting for bloods, having acupuncture, intralipids, obsessing on Google. Time that I could be using growing my business, writing stories, gardening, baking, volunteering.

9. My romantic dream of falling pregnant easily, having a water birth and, in general, just being that irritatingly smug misty-eyed mother you see on 1970s Hallmark cards.

What infertility has given me, AKA the silver lining:

1. Fuck all. Only kidding.

1. Greater empathy for my fellow humans, especially for other women.

2. The realisation that every pregnancy, and every live birth, is nothing short of a miracle.

3. Greater sensitivity in the way I approach other people's problems.

4. The forum has taught me how to care unconditionally: how to listen and support without judgement.

5. A stronger relationship with Mike.

6. Time with the babies at the adoption home. Little munchkins, especially my favourite beloved Crack Baby.

7. Future parenting skills — eventually I will be a better, more patient mother because of this trial, and will never take my baby for granted.

8. A keen vulnerability, like I am balancing on the sharp edge of a knife. I think this will make me a better writer, too.

9. This journal, including the opportunity to make lots of lists.

MOTHER NATURE

Mother Nature

Please forgive me my torn jeans; my bare feet, dirty

My cockiness, my assumed fertility —

My presumption that Life Is Fair.

Please don't forget my cheeky prayers

that lie on the ground

like yesterday's confetti.

DARK WATERFALL

Before I saw Dr Finegan, wonderful Dr Finegan,

the pain was spreading. It was like the shoulder pain was leaking into the rest of my body. Not acute pain, like the source, but a dull ache in my arms and legs. I wondered if it was my body's attempt to get more painkillers — wondered if this is how addiction begins — but then I read a Time magazine article on chronic pain, and it described how pain can 'cascade' into other parts of the body. A dark waterfall. It's some stupid chemical reaction your body has to continual pain. You'd think that years of pain would raise your threshold, but no such luck, according to this report. So much for evolution.

HAVE SEX ALL THE TIME

So, I went to a baby shower today, and I survived. I was feeling brave. I took a bottle of Chardonnay, which helped. I ooh-ed and aah-ed and shared the wine with other reluctant ooh-ers and aah-ers.

I was asked when I was going to 'pop one out' and told them we were about to do our third IVF.

The advice I got to fall pregnant 'naturally' was:

1. Use lots of lube

2. See a Body Talk specialist (WTF?)

3. Have Sex All The Time

I drank my chardonnay. I didn't ovary-act.

Your Story

I read a book the other day about how you must be careful how you tell your story. It certainly applies to me. There is an example of a woman whose husband had cheated on her and her life fell apart after that, and she has this list of things that went wrong after the infidelity and how sad she is now. She carries this list around with her, stapled to her heart, not allowing the good stuff in. The psychologist told her that she needs to forget that story, or at least, her angle on that story. In other words, don't believe everything you think. It is possible to brainwash yourself into a certain state of being — telling yourself you've been cheated by life, or that nobody loves you, or that you're a bad mother, until you see no other reality — you can talk yourself into it, and you can talk yourself out of it. You can change the angle, swap the lens, tell it differently. You can step out of that story.

Knocked Down; Knocked Up

I'm feeling positive today. It's like something clicked in my subconscious, something telling me that I will get my baby, and I feel a sense of peace.

I'm feeling less 'Every time I get up I just get knocked down again' and more 'Every time I get knocked down I just get back up.'

Hopefully soon I will be just plain 'knocked up'.

52

My Haggards

We went for our IVF round 3 briefing with Dr G today. He's concerned that the latest round of stims didn't do much stimulating at all. The blood test results indicate that my ovarian reserve is seriously diminished, and experience tells us that I only have one functioning ovary. Ah, bless my old, haggard ovaries. I would pat them if I could. It's not their fault they've been systematically attacked by endo. Born with a million eggs and all I'm asking is that they do what they were meant to do: just this once. The doc mentioned again that he's worried about the quality of the eggs. I wanted to stick up for them, defend their freshness. 100% fertilisation rate in the first IVF, I wanted to say. Decrepit eggs don't get fertilised. And 2x 5-day embryos. That means they were good quality! But I didn't. I sat there and hugged my babymaker. It's been my one true love/hate relationship.

53

GUINEA PIG

I am to be Dr G's guinea pig. Two supplements, DHEA and Pycnogenal, are going to give my ovaries a bit of a nip and tuck. I picture them now as 70-year-old ladies squeezing and pinching themselves into sequinned dresses that are too small for them, wearing lipstick just a shade too bright, and smiling apologetically at me as if to say: We Are Trying. They will put themselves through the humiliation of being mutton dressed as lamb just this once, this one last chance.

DHEA has been proven (in only one very small study in the US) not only to increase fertility but live birth rates by 300%. Apparently it makes you feel like a teenager again (read: gives you moods and bad skin). I wonder if it'll stall my wrinkling. It would be *kak* unfair to have acne and wrinkles at the same time.

Pycnogenal (pick-nodge-an'all) is the pine bark with *je ne sais quoi*. The champagne of supplements. Difficult to pronounce, even more difficult to find in a pharmacy. But! *S'il vous plaît,* what does it do? *Sacré bleu!* More like, what doesn't it do? This concentrated antioxidant anti-inflammatory can cure anyone of anything. Think snake oil, or, rather, snake sawdust. *Serpent Sciure.*

Both are supposed to help with my egg quality (although I truly don't understand how you can improve egg quality — surely an egg is as fresh as it is, and you can't make it any fresher short of jumping into Doc's time machine like Marty McFly? Where is a flux capacitor when you need one?). I know how powerful the placebo effect can be, so I'm not going to ask too many questions.

Resounding Silence

After my Mike Junior Fan Club update today, about my rotten eggs and being a guinea pig, there was a resounding silence. Usually there is at least a 'Whoo hoo! Holding thumbs!' or a 'Thinking of you guys' or, at the very least, 'Bummer, dude.' But today, nada. I guess it's hard to keep hearing bad news. You run out of positive things to say. Sooner or later you just switch off.

Oh, wait, I spoke too soon. Bing! There is an email from Chris, saying to get him some Pycnogenal, too.

End of the Road

While I have been on the (supplementary) bandwagon, wrecking my skin with abandon and speaking bad French every morning while taking my pine bark, Mike has been less optimistic. In the car on the way home from our last VL appointment he was upset. He thinks that bad egg quality may be the last nail in our fertility coffin. I wondered out loud why he was taking it so hard: why now? We have had so many terrible diagnoses and prognoses along the way that he handled like a seasoned vet. Now he is really sad.

Of course, no one wants to see their favourite person unhappy, and I was sad that he was sad, but a small, secret part of me felt strangely satisfied. At last, I thought, he has realised how serious this is. I felt less lonely. Ashamed, but less lonely.

It's interesting how different people have different take-outs from exactly the same scenario. When Dr G said 'Let's try one last thing,' Mike heard: 'This is most probably the end of the road,' while I heard: 'There is still a chance!' It made me think of those terrible appointments in the beginning when all I heard was: 'You'll never conceive, and if you do, you'll most likely miscarry.' Mike didn't hear the same thing, those many failed cycles ago, and was puzzled by my heartbreak. 'You're acting as if the worst is going to happen,' he said to me, crossly, one day.

Didn't he see? I remember thinking to myself. My greatest fear has been realised. I am infertile. The worst has already happened.

It Works If You Work It

I've been putting off saying this, didn't even want to think it, didn't want to tempt the universe to smack me down again, but I can't keep it in any longer: I think that THE PAIN MEDS ARE WORKING!

Yes, that terrible blue pill (that I sometimes suspected of trying to kill me, that made me so depressed that I started to feel emotionally catatonic) is working. I haven't touched Tramacet or Synap in days. It knocks me out at night. No more fitful sleeping sitting up in bed, no more waking up to a shoulder on fire, no more cracked ribs.

Dare I say it? I think that the Pycnogenal is also helping with the inflammation. I can take deep breaths now, without them shearing through me.

Psychologically I don't feel 100% myself: I sense a distance to my real self, my emotions, which shows in my writing too. The main character in my new novel seems too removed, as if she's sitting on the other side of frosted glass. I'm trying to study her, trying to find the details that will make her real to me and to the reader, but she remains stubbornly aloof. Of course, I'm not so cut off that I don't realise that I, in a way, am her.

This frosted glass, this grey screen, is temporary, I tell myself. And a small price to pay to be able to breathe, to not be in pain.

54

No More Dreaming

I hate it when I'm being realistic about our situation (i.e., saying that my uterus is so toxic that it should have come branded with a skull-and-crossbones) and people chastise me for being negative; but when I'm optimistic ('I think this Pycnogenal is working. Imagine if it works. I mean, really works. IVF round 3 is coming up ... I could be pregnant by Christmas!') then people give me this pitying look, this sorry stare, and tell me not to get my hopes up. Please, people, pick a side.

I am realistic. Or at least, I'm trying to be realistic. I don't need you to be my pinball cushions; I'm perfectly fine smashing into the walls on my own.

Don't tell me 'Just Be Positive!' You know where 'positive thinking' got me? It got me thinking I could wait until I was 30 before trying to start a family. It got me trying to conceive for a whole precious year on my own as the endometriosis insidiously furred over all my organs like malignant moss. It got me trying 'natural therapies' and a kind giant of a doctor who wasted another precious year with his ancient x-ray machine and turkey baster and just-off-the-mark diagnosis. It got be heartbroken over a first IVF, depressed after a second. It got me to 32 with old eggs and a wasted-away babymaker. Fuck Positive Thinking. Positive Thinking sets you up for month after month of disappointment and despair. It's not healthy. I'm much better off without it. Sometimes it seems as there is no light at the end of the birth canal.

ANOTHER REASON TO NOT BELIEVE IN GOD

Today there was someone in the forum who had three IVFs, every one of them ending in miscarriages. During the third pregnancy they lost their twin girls at 21 weeks. While the woman was stimming for her fourth IVF her husband was shot and killed in a hijacking. I have no words.

...

I've just realised that I've stopped dreaming. The blue pills. Nights have turned into long dark slabs of unconsciousness.

GIANT GREEN PHONE

Got the call from Dr G today that we can go ahead with our third and final IVF. The blood results weren't promising, but the markers were sufficiently in-range to begin stimming. After three months of being on DHEA and Pycnogenal, my oestrogen had come down significantly (good news), but my other numbers showed little improvement and the doc isn't happy, which scares the shitkittens out of me. On the phone I was, like, low ovarian reserve? We knew that already. We've had this conversation before. It's like *deja vu*, except that this time I picture him at his desk like a captain in a control room, with his hand hovering over the big red button. Holy shit, I think — cold, but sweating — how did I let this get away from me? What have I done? Why didn't we pull out the big guns sooner, when we still had something to work with? But then he makes a small joke, says something mildly optimistic, and then I can breathe again. Now I picture him talking into a giant green phone. So we're going ahead? I ask. Affirmative, he says. We're going ahead.

...

I texted Mike about Dr G on the giant green phone. He replied: 'Let's give it all we've got. I'll start doing push-ups again.'

CLAPPING

Today there was an article in the New York Times about how everyday stress is not linked to infertility. Oh, how I wanted to shout it from the rooftops. There was a festive atmosphere on the forum: the girls had circulated the article far and wide. At last, we said, evidence. A legitimate study. At last our friends and family would stop believing the myth that if we 'just relaxed' then 'it would happen'.

What did you say, strange lady at the party with watery eyes and wobbly chin? Science isn't enough for you? You still think I should just calm the fuck down about it? You still think that if I stopped focussing on my dream of having a baby that my endo would magically disappear and that my ovaries would un-wilt and be so brimming with beautiful, ripe eggs that they would start clapping? Maybe chest-bumping each other? Come closer, cheap-gold crucifix-clutching lady, tell me about that friend-of-a-friend you know that fell pregnant after adopting. And that other friend-of-a-friend, your cousin's best friend's father's sister, that 'gave up' and 'stopped trying,' only to find that she was pregnant with twins. Come here, strange lady. Put down that chip-and-dip and let me high-five your face.

55

SLIPPERIEST OF SLOPES

I've never been obsessed with money. If I had been I would have chosen to be a chartered accountant instead of an art director (and then a book dealer and writer). I don't see wealth as a measure of consummate success. I'm a seriously low maintenance girl and get by easily without feeling that I am missing out, as long as I have my basic wants and needs met (Mike, friends and family, cats, house in Parkhurst, garden, unit trusts, books, laptop, passport, wine). I've been driving the same (sunburnt, bumped, ever-loyal) car for 12 years. I still colour my own hair, for heaven's sake (#firstworldproblems). I marvel at beauty features in magazines when the writer describes her new favourite make-up for the month. For the *month*? It takes me a year to go through my one stick of eyeliner.

I'd rather have fewer things and more meaning.

Don't get me wrong. Obviously I'd like to have more cash — who wouldn't? — but I'm not sure I'd be terribly good at spending it, apart from travelling more. In fact, one of my biggest life lessons about money/happiness came from travelling.

When I was 18 I au-paired for a wonderful Swiss / German family in Lörrach, Germany. We lived on the border of France and Switzerland, and neither of the parents were working and they were properly loaded, so we basically spent the year travelling. It was one of the most amazing experiences I've ever had, and I still think of them often and with much love. One of the highlights (there were many — enough to write a book about) was flying to Paris for a weekend. It was my first time and it was spectacular. We stayed in an amazing hotel and ate at one of the best restaurants in the city: up in the Eiffel Tower. I tried *cuisses de grenouille* and everything from beginning to end was incredible.

A few months later, on break from the au-pairing, Pin, Pom and I went backpacking through Germany, Holland, France and England. We also stopped in Paris (how could we not?) but we couldn't afford accommodation. We walked and walked all night, taking it in. We stumbled upon an aviation street exhibition. We had dinner at a steakhouse (*steak! pommes frites! vin rouge!*), dragging the meal out for hours to take advantage of the warmth and light, the soft seats, until we were the last table and reluctantly took leave. When the sun started rising and the street washers came with their hoses we ducked into a McDonalds bathroom to brush our teeth.

Five-star Paris with my host parents was wonderful and I'll never forget it as long as I live, but Paris with my closest friends, despite being poor, dirty backpackers, was better.

But now I find myself money-hungry. I feel like the fertility treatments drain every cent that I have, and more. We keep taking more and more hard-earned cash out of the bond, and the debt is gnawing at my stomach, snapping at my heels like an especially frisky Jack Russell. We need to decide on some kind of cap before everything is gone.

The thing about assisted reproduction is that it is the slipperiest of slopes. You go from certainly, absolutely, not doing fertility treatments, to just doing a medicated cycle, to just doing IUI, to doing 'just one round' of IVF. It's like someone who disapproves of gambling buying a Lotto ticket, then being shown the slot machine, then having a go at the poker table. Next thing you know, you've lost your car, your house, and your engagement ring in a particularly brutal game in the casino's VIP lounge where the drinks are free. Sometimes you win, most of the time you don't. Most of the time it's a game of trading up and up and up until you look down and there's nothing under your feet, like the coyote who runs off the cliff in Roadrunner.

56

IVF #3

Thundercats Are Go!

Third time lucky. Third time lucky. Third time lucky. Right?

Going in for the first scan tomorrow. Mike doesn't bother coming to these scans anymore. What's the point? If I could skip them too, I would. Send my uterus in via courier and hope it doesn't get stuck in traffic, or lost on the way back.

In our first cycle of IVF we hoped for between 8 and 12 follicles, and we got 7. It was probably due to my poor ovarian reserve and the fact that I seem to have only one mildly enthusiastic ovary. This time we are hoping for the best in a bad situation, as we know that reserve has since halved. While we are hoping for lucky number 7 again, we will be overjoyed at any number over 3 (under 4 and the cycle gets cancelled, like last time). Dr G has upped my Menopur from 5 amps a day to 6 (regular dose is 3) to get my stubborn haggards to up their game.

We've got so much stacked up against us, it's difficult to be optimistic, but knowing that this is our last IVF brings with it equal measures of desperation and acceptance, and I oscillate between the two. Again I am doing everything I can to make it work: monkey diet / reflexology / acupuncture / hypnosis / intralipids, although I have stopped praying. I don't see the point. Instead I am numbly going through the motions, like a whipped dog doing tricks.

HANGRY FOR HEADS

Trying to not lose my shit today. Along with gift vouchers, VL should offer an Anger Management class.

Today, it was the doctors who pissed me off especially.

1. Dr V, while scanning me on CD2, looked at my uterus and said that there was 'too much blood' to start our IVF today. WTF? Of course there is lots of blood. It's the second day of my period! So I woke up at 4:30am to get here by 5:30am to be told that there is a lot of blood in my full-steam-ahead-menstruating uterus. Awesome. See you same time tomorrow, then.

2. Dr G. When we were discussing the protocol, I told him about the pain medication I was on and he said I should 'be careful'. Really, doc? Because usually I'm so careless with my health? Because I'm tossing schedule 6s

down my throat without a thought of how it will affect my body and my fertility? Because I'm taking chronic meds that depress me, that switch my brain off, just for shits and giggles? It occurs to me that he has never understood the magnitude of my pain.

Have I entered the Angry Stage? Or is it the hormones making me so prickly? Whatever the reason, if anyone around me manages to keep their head on their shoulders lately they should consider themselves 'lucky'. I'm hangry for heads. I'm like the Queen of Hearts (uterus-shaped hearts?) in Wonderland, marching around shouting 'Off with his head! Off with her head!' except that I don't want my card-soldiers to do the beheading — I want to bite them off myself.

HUNGOVER(Y)

Calmer today, but not great news. This morning's scan showed that my ovaries are still recovering from our last cycle. We were told there was no problem in doing-back-to-back IVF cycles, but apparently there is. Who knew that an ovary could get a hangover? Understandably, the doc didn't want to sweatshop it by pumping it full of stimulation drugs.

So, in an ironic twist, I am on the pill for 15 days, to calm it down. Yes, that pill. Contraception. Ha ha. Ha, ha, universe, ha, ha.

57

IVF #3 TAKE 2

And ... here we go again. IVF #3 take 2. I can almost hear the clapperboard snap in my brain.

...

Usually at this point in stimming I am in agony and taking my maximum dosage (and more) of painkillers, but the Trepiline is keeping the knife at bay — or at least, just the tip is embedded in my shoulder, instead of the whole hot length. Dare I hope that this cycle will have a different outcome because I am not writhing in pain?

HITCHING UP MY SKIRT

You have to take the Menopur at a certain time every day and we weren't close to home, so we had to shoot up in the public toilet in a hospital this morning. Oh, how my life has changed, I thought, not for the first time. Mike sneaking into the Ladies behind me; me hitching up my skirt and bending over. No kissing, no heavy breathing, just cold white tiles and the assailing smell of antiseptic gel and pink toilet freshener. After a difficult morning it was decidedly UNfunny but we laughed anyway, which, I am sure, didn't make us look any more innocent as we tiptoed our way out of there.

...

Our stimming didn't go very well: we have 4 follicles. 6 amps of Menopur a day and all we got were 4 lousy follies. Not ideal, not even good, but enough not to cancel the cycle, and at this stage we will take what we can get. It's tough, but we're coping.

Sometimes, on a day like today, I'm feeling fine one moment — even happy. But then the bad-news infertility monster rears up, Python-like, and strikes me on the hand.

I cried today, over the 4 follies. 'Cried' may be an understatement. How will we have a chance if we've got so little to work with? I thought I was okay with it, I took the news well in the scanning room, tried to 'Be Positive!' but it turned out I was just in denial. In truth, of course, I wasn't crying over the follies but everything it has taken to get to this point. All along I've been pulled in and further in by the tide and now the huge wave has crashed over me.

When Mike saw me crying he got angry. Demanded to know why I was so upset; why I was acting like it was over. There is so much riding on this cycle; I just needed a release. It's a stressful time for both of us, I understand that he needs a release too, but he shouldn't have bullied me. And then I got angry at him getting angry, and cried more. I feel like he pounced on me today, at my most vulnerable. Don't think I've ever felt this lonely.

WHY YOU WERE TAKEN

I'm distracting myself this month by working on my new novel. It's about a red-haired synaesthete with 'bad habits and a fertility problem'. Sound familiar? While she is kind of me, she's not me at all. She's bad-ass. It's set in near-future Jo'burg. It's called 'Why You Were Taken'.

...

Holy Moses, I am so bored of intralipids. Today, feeling exhausted, I gave up my ruse of wounded receptionist at the front desk and instead grabbed a lazy chair right at the back and ploughed my way through the latest Marian Keyes. I needed something undemanding and funny, something that would make the hours of waiting for blood test results and scans and soya oil drips fly by. It worked. I almost wanted the IV to take longer than it did.

It's in my nature to squeeze as much working time out of the day as I can. I work all day and most week nights. When you work for yourself and you love your job it's easy to fall into the trap of working all the time. I like being constructive. If I'm not working, I'm writing. There always seems to be a project that I'm not spending quite enough time on. And then there is the house and the hobbies: gardening, reading, running, walking, yoga. There are never enough hours in the day for what I want to get done. That's why I usually bring my laptop to the clinic and hammer away at my keyboard like a chimpanzee on speed. It's not that I don't know how to let my hair down, believe me, I do. I think I would have done well in the '80s corporate world: Work Hard, Play Hard. Martinis at lunch.

But lately I've been missing so much work with the surgeries and the treatments and the downtime that I have to make it up somehow if I want my business to survive. Infertility has leached so much from me, it will not claim my sweat-and-blood business.

So I did take my laptop in, as always, and was greeted by the smirking nurses, as always, but then I thought, Fuck It. I'm tired. Today I'm reading. And then I saw the tea and rusks and thought, Fuck It. Fuck the monkey diet. Fuck it all. And I curled up on a chair with my tea and my Marian Keyes and it was four hours of absolute luxury. When is the last time I had four hours of uninterrupted reading time? When is the last time anyone had four hours of uninterrupted reading time? When they removed the drip I waltzed out of there like I had just had a mini-vacation. From now on, unless I have something that is very urgent to attend to, and especially if there are no martinis on hand, I will be leaving my laptop snug it its bag and reading my way through the rest of these appointments.

58

Plot Twist

My scan today was to monitor the progress of the four follicles. The dildo cam is whipped out in all its lubed glory and the big black dots on the screen are measured to within a millimetre of their short lives. Once they reach a certain size they are deemed mature and ready to harvest, like sun-ripened grapes (if you were to harvest grapes by knocking someone out and then plunging a long needle up their vajayjay). It sounds painful, but really all it entails is (another) day off work and some lovely anaesthetic.

It's not just junkie-me that enjoys the anaesthetic: the girls on the forum are forever saying: 'Good luck and enjoy the drugs!' when someone is going in for egg retrieval, as if they are going off to Burning Man or something.

On Saturday the doc didn't even bother scanning my left (AKA lazy-ass) ovary because in the 2+ years of scans and treatments it has never ovulated. Slacker!

Sometimes we can't even make out the actual ovary, as if it has teleported its way out of my hopeless babymaker to go and do something more useful somewhere else.

Poor smoker's ovary on the right hand side has had to do all the work, despite its sorry state. It's probably tired of being sweat-shopped by Menopur. No wonder it had that cyst: a psychosomatic symptom of a nervous breakdown. How else could it tell us? We don't speak Ovary. It's clearly burnt out and we just keep flogging it like a dying camel.

But then this morning the doc glimpsed the perpetual slacker and was, like, 'Whoah! What's that?'

Leftie has decided to come to the IVF party with two mature follies (and two smaller ones) which means that we have SIX mature follies, maybe even seven, which is almost double what we thought we had before. I don't know what happened but I am doing a rain-dance-like gratitude shimmy to the DHEA and magical pine bark gods, just in case they had something to do with it. And Leftie! Leftie who decided that now is the time to shine up. Don't get me started. I am high-fiving him every chance I get.

I was kind of pretending that I thought we had a shot with only four follies (what else could I do?) but now I really think we have a chance. A real chance.

...

The pain is back.

Couldn't sleep last night. I thought we'd got it under control, but it seems that even Trepiline is no match for 6 amps of Menopur a day. I've been popping pills like

Smarties, trying not to complain too much. Keeping my eyes on the prize.

We're 'growing' the follies for a few more days before retrieval. I just need to make it till then.

. . .

A tender moment I'll never forget: One night when I was feeling sad about our fertility prognosis, Mike and I were sitting together at the dining room table. There wasn't much more to say so we sat still for a while, in silence, and he put his bare foot under mine. It was warm and it meant: This is going to be okay.

UFO

Scan and bloods went well this morning. I am being especially nice to my left ovary for her last-ditch effort. I'll be going in for retrieval in a couple of days.

Dr G was pleased with my trilaminar endometrial lining. In peasant-speak, this is a certain way lining can present that looks like three lines: what the doc calls a flying saucer, or UFO. Like alien conspiracy theorists, they don't see it as often as they'd like to.

'This is really good,' he said. 'This is really good,' he said again, which made me a little bit excited. I had never even heard of the flying saucer. Was the UFO like some kind of hush-hush privilege of an undisclosed society, like the secret menu at Starbucks? I couldn't wait to tell the girls on the forum.

...

Absolutely thrilled to wake up after ER to see a sticker on my hand reading: '10 eggs. Well done! (:'

TEN EGGS!!!!!!!! Where did they come from?

I know that some of them will be immature, but look at that number. Isn't it wonderful?

F U N E X? V F X! V F 10 X!

...

Got the embryologist's call at 8:30 this morning: 6 eggs fertilised and they're 'looking great'. 3 of the 10 were immature and one fertilised abnormally, so it won't survive. We have 6 embryos! 6! The most fertile number there is.

She'll call again tomorrow morning with a progress report. If they are not looking as strong tomorrow then we'll have a 3-day transfer, but we're hoping to go to 5 days (near blastocyte stage), as blasts have a better chance of implanting. Grow, little embies, grow!

...

5 of our embryos made it through the night, with 3 taking the lead with 6 cells each, and the other 2 slowly doing their thing at 4 cells. They gave us a print-out of the pictures of the babies. Absolutely amazing. One is the shape of a rugby ball — I'm sure it must be a boy? The doc, perhaps concerned about the slowing of the 2, has recommended that we do a 3-day transfer tomorrow

morning. Ack! So I've got the IL IV in as I write, and trying to get all my work done while I wait, so that I can take the whole day off tomorrow. Also need to squeeze in another session of acupuncture and hypnosis today, if I can. So I'm quoting and processing orders but I feel a bit light-headed because the doc couldn't find a vein in my hand and I watched the needle threading in and out a couple of times. Woozy, but, looking at the picture of our embryos, optimistic. They'll be back on the mothership tomorrow, and that makes me happy.

I asked the Mike Jnr Fan Club how many embryos they think we should back, and the replies were unanimous: ALL OF THEM.

Mike and I have spoken about it at length, and are leaning towards three. Last time we put two healthy-looking 5-day embryos back, and got nothing. Now we have three goodies and a UFO. We're up for twins. Hell, at this stage, we're even up for triplets. I'm not sure Dr G will let us transfer that many. This is our last chance.

GREY CLOUD

We were sitting in the clinic waiting room, waiting to be called for transfer, when we got called into Dr V's office (it felt exactly like being called into the headmaster's office). Our first and only thoughts were: Oh, Fuck.

I was sure that he would open the door for us with a pained, if not polite, smile; motion to seats with a grey cloud for a face. Say that he's not sure what happened, but all the embryos had died overnight.

Instead, there was good news. He said that the two slow-growers had been pacing themselves to wow us on day 3. Now we have FIVE really good embryos again and it's impossible to say which are the strongest, so we're going to do a 5-day transfer. It took a while to take this in.

...

We went to Ben's first birthday party today. He was just too sweet. How I love that boy! After we sang happy birthday to him he clapped for us. Heart = melted. Pin made an amazing cake topped with zoo animals. Flings were eaten. Everyone was kind to me, no one offered unsolicited advice.

Ex-boyfriend B was there. He is dating a seriously lovely girl that we've known for ages. They look good together. People say that the only real revenge you need on your ex is to be happy and successful, and if that is true then I consider him avenged. And maybe I am now taking too much for granted, but perhaps I am forgiven. At the very least, we both know that what we had was genuine. How else would we be able to sincerely wish for each other's happiness?

It was difficult to relax. No matter how much I tried to be in the moment, my mind would wander to my five little embabies in the lab. I ran after kids and made small talk and served ice cream from a million miles away.

I am now less than a day away from being pregnant, or never being pregnant at all. If it weren't for the Trepiline I'd probably lie awake all night with the sheer terror and wonder of it.

59

SEND IN THE CLOWNS

There is something that happens in an embryo sometime between day 3 and day 5 where a 'switch' is turned on (or not) and the cell becomes self-sufficient (or not), so transferring on day 5 means that you can make a much more informed decision on which ones to put back, and the success rates are higher. Alternative thought is that a petri dish is no place for any living thing, not really, and the best place by far is where the embryo should have been in the first place, being kept snug in mama's velvety lining. I'm chuffed about getting to day 5: I think the stronger the baba can get before being transported to my extraterrestrial uterus, the better.

In our pre-transfer chat with Dr G I was prepared to try to persuade him to let us put three embryos back. I had been practising my speech in the car, on the way to the clinic. I had all my points lined up. I was ready. After he showed us more updated pics of the babies and we cooed accordingly, I asked him how many he would recommend, and he said 'Three!' without hesitation. Tables turned, I asked him if he was sure. 'Absolutely,' he said, 'Three is our lucky number.' I felt relieved and nervous in equal measure.

The transfer went really well, with smiles and high-fives all round. I don't remember the staff being that happy after IVF #1. A beetle of paranoia scuttled over me: had they known something during that last transfer that we didn't? And made us wait that torturous two weeks anyway? But there was no use in thinking about that now.

Also: a moment before the celebratory atmosphere erupted we had a moment of near-catastrophe. I had been reading about how to up the success rate of IVF (no surprise there) and came across a study done in Israel where the fertility specialist arranged for a 'medical clown' to make the women undergoing IVF laugh, to excellent results. I question this study of only 219 women because it was so small but more importantly: what the fuck is a 'medical clown'? Just the thought of that scares the hell out of me. How do they know that it was the so-called 'laughing' and not the utter horror of seeing such a thing, that made the difference? A clown is scary enough (Hello? Does no one read Stephen King?) but one in scrubs, snapping latex gloves, makes me want to screw my eyes shut and call for my happy place (and a change of underwear).

Anyway, I once again put my reservations aside (I now believe in magic, see?) and briefed Mike to make me laugh as much as he could on the morning of transfer. I had funny videos pre-loaded on my phone. We reminded each other of funny stories. When the time came, we cast around for VL clowns and were relieved to find none (they were probably hiding under my hospital bed), and so it was up to Mike to tell me jokes. I was nervous as hell, giddy (hysterical?), so the laughs came easily. I wasn't sure exactly when I should be laughing, pre- or post-transfer, so I figured I would just laugh all along. Of course, I had to remember not to laugh too hard (you have to have a full bladder for the procedure) and I didn't want to literally piss myself laughing. Having five people look up your punani at the same time is humiliating enough.

It was going according to plan until the actual transfer took place. The embryologist made Mike check that they were loading the correct embryos into the syringe (our surname was engraved into the petri dish glass) and when he had confirmed and come back to my side (dim room, legs in stirrups) and they started threading the catheter, ready to inject the precious cargo into my babymaker, Mike murmured: 'It would have been awkward if they'd mixed them up.' When I frowned at him for an explanation, he said: 'The other two dishes were Naidoo and Tshabalala.'

I guffawed at exactly the wrong time, and Dr G yelled 'Hold still!' as if it were life or death (of course it was life or death) and then I froze and held my breath and the babies were in and we could exhale. Everyone in the room seemed really pleased, acting as if I was already pregnant, patting themselves and us, on the back, and we couldn't help but leave with grins on our faces.

They gave us a print-out of the sonar, showing a little flash of light, like a shooting star, of the moment the embryos were transferred. How amazing would it be to show that to the triplets one day?

Okay, so I know the chances of triplets are less than 1%, but I can't help thinking of my three embabies as just that. The Lawrence triplets are on board! Isn't it wonderful to think that they are inside me now? I've been speaking to them and eating ice cream and generally trying to make them feel at home. I'm officially PUPO (Pregnant Until Proven Otherwise).

...

I've been cooing over the pictures of the embryos, and sent them to pretty much everyone in my entire address book. I have the shot on my phone, too, to show random strangers. I don't know if I'll ever get to be that person with pictures of their kids in their wallets, so I'm jumping on this for now. Aren't they just beautiful? I say. The one shaped like a rugby ball must be a boy, I quip, over and over again, to different people. I think I must have a mad glint in my eye.

...

I've been so nice to the triplets. We went for a walk in the sunshine yesterday, and then last night I didn't feel like running or going to yoga so we skipped gym and watched a funny movie instead. I've been on the lookout for any sign of implantation, but *nada*. I wish I could feel SOMETHING but I still enjoy the knowledge that I might be preggo. Mike is being kind and supportive and I feel very much in love with him. We're not allowed to do the diggety. My womb has to be free from original sin. I'm sure blow jobs don't count. Maybe that's what Mary said.

SURVIVOR

We went out for dinner with Mandie and Avish last night. Their support throughout this nightmare has been unparalleled. They have been there for us from (even before) the very beginning. They were right by our side during those first few months of awkward expectation, bolstering our hope when it became clear that we had a problem, and pouring me large whiskies throughout the nitty-gritties of devil wombs and angry vaginas. Now, almost three years later, they sit across from us at a homely Italian place in Parkview, with me urging them to drink my share of wine. The food was simple, warm, delicious, the conversation comforting.

Walking to the car afterwards, cheeks bitten pink by the cold, Mandie said something about it working this time. It'll be a survivor, she says. I had been lulled by the easy evening, I dropped my guard.

If anything manages to live in my toxic uterus it will most certainly be a survivor, I said, it's killed off everything else. Her mouth hung open. How can you say that?

Easily, I shrugged. It's true.

...

I was standing at the kitchen counter, making tea as meditatively as possible, when I felt the slightest, vaguest hint of something in my uterus. A twitch. A scrape. Like someone had given me the most gentle scratchy poke with a knitting needle. And then it was gone. Holy shit, I thought to myself, oh holy shit, was that implantation? Was that one of the trips burrowing in? Of course it probably wasn't, and I have been driven to delusion by this two-week wait, but can you imagine if I do get the Big Fat Positive? I will be able to recall this mind-blowing moment when I felt my baby stick.

60

RABBIT HOLE

I cracked. I know it was a terrible idea, but I POASed today and the test was negative. Big Fat Fucking Negative.

9DP5DT (9 days post 5 day transfer): 2 days to go till my official blood test and no shoulder pain (yet), and I just couldn't wait an hour longer. So the torturous anticipation has been replaced by a full-body numb kind of dread. I can't believe this has happened. I'm angry at the world and at myself for being stupid and naïve enough to believe that I could get pregnant in the first place. Every single thing that has happened in this IF 'journey' (fuck the word 'journey'. That's like calling a trip to hell a 'journey') has pointed to one outcome, and I was too damned dewy-eyed to realise it. This is where 'positive thinking' gets you: to the bottom of a deep, dark hole: broke and broken. Broken in every way. I hate it, I hate it, I hate everything.

I wanted to smash things. I wanted to rage around the house and scoop anything that could shatter onto the floor. I wanted to kick down doors and punch windows. Instead I sat at the kitchen table, evil stick in hand, with a blank look on my face. Bereft.

'Maybe it's too early to test,' ventured Mike.

'Maybe the sticks are too old to work properly,' I said, stroking the dusty packaging.

Where is that huge box of bulk pregnancy tests that should be in every infertile's cupboard? Ah, fuck, I think, there I go again. Scratching, scrabbling, scavenging for hope like a starving chicken on a landfill. Or a land-mine.

My world has fallen around me. I didn't know what to do with myself. I couldn't stay in the house. I plugged in my music, pulled on my Nikes and went for a long, long run. I hadn't run in two weeks — since the transfer — and it felt good. Running stopped me from crying. I'm all for crying: it's the healthiest way to release your emotions, etc. etc., but I thought that if I started I would never stop. I'd be like the Forrest Gump of criers: I would weep for days, for weeks, for years. Journalists would show up outside our house, wanting to interview me, but they wouldn't be able to make out what I was saying through the impressive stamina of my *snot en trane*. They would give up, eventually, but leave behind their Energades and bottled water, worried at how I would stay hydrated.

...

I sent the update to the Mike Jnr Fan Club, and posted my BFN on the forum. So much love and support. If the treatment had worked this little baby would have had such an amazing circle of love.

We put back three very healthy looking embryos. THREE! How can I possibly be that broken?

I can't believe that I have lost the triplets. I had bonded with each of them. All the love, time, effort, money spent on this cycle, down the drain. What hurts most is, after 26 negative cycles in a row, the dreadful, dreadful feeling that I'll never conceive.

Mike and I have started talking about our POA (but what is left to try?) and will wait till we see our doc before we make any decisions. In the meantime, I am trying not to think at all.

...

My dad emailed back: 'What's a POA?!' (Most likely wondering what I am peeing on now.)

Plan Of Action, Dad, I wrote back.

THE PLOT (WIP)

1. Wedding! Honeymoon! Off the pill! So excited! Life is Awesome!

...

28. Decide to do one last round of IVF. 3rd time lucky?

29. IVF #3 BFN.

30. The End. Condemned to being a childless mother.

31. No, wait, hang on. What about egg donation?

...

It's late at night, too late. It feels like the last night before the rest of my life. I will be a different person tomorrow. I will have resigned myself to being a barren piece of junk. I don't know when acceptance will come.

Mike and I have been smashing our heads against the great wall of infertility. When do you call it quits? When is giving up the right thing to do? We have gotten this far down the rabbit hole because of my dogged insistence, my desperation to realise my life's dream. I don't regret it, despite my scars. I knew that I had to try absolutely everything or risk regretting it the rest of my life.

My breastbone is tender: literal heartache. I don't know if I can live this life. Someone got it wrong. This is not the life for me.

...

I'm at the bottom of the hole, the damp, smelly well, when Mike said: 'Well, what's next? What else can we do?'

Nothing, I wanted to say. Nothing. It's over. We're all out of options, but that wasn't true.

'We could use someone else's eggs,' I said, not quite believing it, finding the idea completely bizarre (but not more bizarre, I reasoned later, than a 'test-tube baby').

'How do you do that?' Mike asked. I shrugged, and Googled it. There are two well-respected agencies that arrange egg donation in South Africa, and I scour their websites. It's like online dating. You get to search via location, hair colour, eye colour, tertiary education, interests, medical history. There are pages and pages of pretty women staring back at me. Most of them have completed their family and want to help infertile couples conceive. What kind of person sells their eggs, we wonder. Overly-kind people, and overly-desperate-for-cash people. Oh, this one looks nice, I say to Mike. She likes reading, and books. She looks a bit like me, if you kind of squint sideways at the screen. More like, if you close your eyes, Mike says. What about this one? She seems beautiful and clever. No chronic diseases in her family. Why didn't we go this route to begin with? I joke. This chick's DNA is way better than mine!

There is evidence, says one of the websites, that the DNA of the pregnant woman determines the expression of the donor-egg baby's genes. In other words, the baby gets her genes from the sperm and the egg donor, but the 'instructions' on how to activate them come from the woman who carries her. So, in essence, the baby has three biological parents. It's called epigenetics. Sci-fi enough for you?

They give an example of horse-breeding, where it is not uncommon to implant a pony embryo in the womb of a horse. The foals that result are bigger than regular ponies. Their genotype is the same as a pony's but their phenotype (the expression of their genes) is different. I gave Mike a quick rundown of the theory of epigenetics, citing the pony/horse example, as we flicked through mugshots.

That one looks a bit horsey, he said.

We continued looking at prospective donors for a while, rating them as if we were judges on American Idol. That's a NO from me, Mike said, looking at a woman with too many teeth in her mouth. All of a sudden we had some small measure of control again (even if it was imagined), and we both felt a bit better. The good news is that maybe we're not completely out of options, although we're not really sure that this is a viable alternative. How far is too far? And, more importantly, why would someone else's egg survive in my chamber of death if our five beautiful embryos didn't? The bad news is that a donor egg cycle costs double that of a regular IVF, and we've already spent R200,000 using our access bond as a credit card. Buying an *actual horse* may be cheaper than getting our grubby hands on a couple of eggs. I consider pawning my engagement ring.

If a kid ever does come along I hope he doesn't mind eating cat food for the foreseeable future.

61

COULD IT POSSIBLY BE TRUE?

This morning my shoulder was still suspiciously pain-free so I decided to pee on a(nother) evil stick. Knowing that it would be negative I put it down on the kitchen table and carried on reading my book. Horrible thing, I thought, it didn't deserve another second of my attention.

Mike had made us fresh juice earlier (carrot, cucumber, apple, ginger) and he joked that the juice was so good it would trick the stick into giving us a positive. He walked past the table, also kind of giving the test the silent treatment, the averted gaze, when he said softly: 'There's a faint line.'

What do you mean, there's a faint line? WHAT DO YOU MEAN THERE IS A FAINT LINE? I didn't believe him until I had the stick in my hands and saw the double lines, and then I still didn't believe I was pregnant. The test was old; expired. Not worth the pee that had landed on it.

'There's a faint line,' Mike had said. We looked at each other in silence as the impossible sunk in. There was no happy dance, no joyful yelling, no high-fiving. We sat down on the couch, thighs touching, elbows on knees, and both bawled our eyes out. You'd swear that someone had just told us that our entire family has been wiped out by a freak accident, so very ugly was our ugly cry. We sobbed for ages, until there was nothing left. Then we hugged and smiled and hugged some more. I imagined that the overriding emotion would be joy, but really it was relief. A huge warm gush of relief. Was the nightmare over?

Of course, we couldn't stake our claim on the future like that on an ancient stick of evil. We needed confirmation. Pregnancy tests had been improved in the three years since I had bought this old one. Now clever digital ones are available. Mike was out the door before I could say 'Clearblue'. I drank more juice. I told myself not to count my chickens. POASing was one thing, a blood test was another. Getting through the first trimester was not guaranteed. I told myself not to count my chickens but they were tapping their way out of their shells like crazed storks.

Mike got back holding the pharmacy's paper bag like a World Cup trophy. I've never been so excited to pee in my life. The result was almost immediate: 2–3 WEEKS PREGNANT.

Now the joy started coming, a tide of happiness, a slow, tentative thrill that zipped through me. Now we were laughing, albeit nervously.

How life can change in an instant, I thought. Years ago in the BFG's office, that short moment when I switched from a fertile innocent to damaged goods. Walked in without a pessimistic thought, walked out a different person.

This morning I woke up to the rest of my life as childless, and now ... could I even dare to think it, to say it out loud? And now I have a small embryo(s?!) growing inside me. It feels like a dream. Please God don't let it be a dream.

I phoned Pin in the UK and we celebrated over the phone. I called my Mom and she started crying. My Dad and Gill, my brother. Everyone was fizzing. We floated to Mike's mom, B's, house and told her the news. She didn't believe us. I had to jam the test into her hand. Not strictly sanitary, but in the moment it was forgiven. Mandie and Avish also had to wait to hear it in person; we had a picnic with them at the Emmerentia rose garden later that afternoon. I could tell that they, after my bleak update the day before, had all their cheering points worked out: ready to make me feel better, and when we told them that everything had changed they were momentarily dumbstruck, and then they slowly warmed to cautious delight. They, more than anyone, knew the risks, knew the stakes. They had seen me at my lowest, in my emotional gutter. They had held my decaying zombie hand.

We all lay quietly in the dappled light, under a massive oak tree. We sipped gingerbeer and spoke of a gentle future. Something big and dark had shifted, and although it had left an indelible footprint, we were at last able to glimpse the light.

On the drive home, Mike put his hand on my knee.

'Being pregnant feels like Christmas,' he said. 'Everyone is happy.'

...

Oh my HAT still waiting for a beta! I was knocking on the door at 6:55AM asking for a blood test. Two hours later they still haven't called. I've phoned VL about 20 times in the last 20 minutes.

...

Beta finally in. 327. When I answered the phone I think I managed to send a stream of rainbows darting into the nurse's ear. She said: 'It sounds like you already know the result,' and I said: 'I peed on a stick.' And she said 'Congratulations.'

(I think she meant for falling pregnant, not for peeing on a stick.)

The girls on the forum have been amazing: stoking my excitement, soothing my fears. I still feel like I'm dreaming. Still don't believe it 100%. I'm going for another beta on Wednesday, and if my beta has doubled, another dose of intralipids. We need to keep this baby on board. If a 3rd beta on Friday is again doubled, the pregnancy is confirmed. The next hurdle is our first scan at seven weeks. SEVEN WEEKS? I have to wait another three weeks to see my babba? To hear his heartbeat, to know that he is real. I can't believe I am lucky enough to be even be thinking of my baby's heartbeat. There is a baby. There is a baby. There is a baby.

...

Facebook status update:

1x IVP, 2x HSG, 2x IUIs, 1x laparoscopy, 3x hysteroscopies, 3x medicated cycles, endless timed cycles, 3x IVFs and one big, beautiful BFP.

62

WOMB OF DOOM

Waiting for the first scan is torture. The two-week-wait is nothing compared to this. The statistics are that as many as 50% of pregnancies end in miscarriage. IVF pregnancies are more at risk than unassisted pregnancies. Of those 50%, most will occur before the woman even knows she is pregnant. She will bleed normally and never guess that she had conceived. It's called a chemical pregnancy or a 'missed pregnancy'.

Getting a BFP is the first hurdle. If you can get past CD28, you have passed the second hurdle. If you get to hear the heartbeat at 7/8/9 weeks, then the third hurdle can eat your dust. Every hurdle you skim not only gets you closer to the finish line, but increases your odds of getting there. If you can make it through the first rocky trimester, you are (almost) out of the woods. If you can make it past the second trimester there is a very good chance your baby will survive. Dr G goes further than this and says that it's only really a sure thing when the kid turns 1.

As I said, waiting to hear the heartbeat is torture. I'm trying to 'Just Be Positive!!!' and I do find myself floating on Cloud 9 most of the day (waking up pain-free and pregnant), but there is the nagging worry that my Chamber of Doom is, well, a Chamber of Doom. Womb of Doom.

My current thinking is that infertility has already taken so much from me, that I'm not going to let it take my excitement and joy in these first fragile three months. Sure, I need to be realistic, but I will not say 'IF we have a baby in 8 months ...' or 'IF this pregnancy works out' ... Instead I'm saying 'I'M HAVING A BABY!'

I'm going to have a baby. Isn't that amazing?! My biggest dream come true. I am prepared to handle the emotional consequences if it doesn't work, but I'm going to try not to live in trepidation for the next few months. This is most certainly the first and only time I will ever be pregnant, and I'm going to experience all the joy there is to be had for as long as it lasts. In my mind, this baby/ies will be here in April next year. And if we lose them before then, I will deal with it then.

...

2nd beta: 647! That's almost double. That's good enough. No symptoms apart from being really tired. I am weaning myself off the Trepiline so that may have something to do with it.

UPDATE: 3rd beta 1579. More than double. Yay! Do I have more than a singleton inside me? The girls on the forum think so. Their money is on twins. I've already put on 2kg so at least it would be an excuse.

My reflexologist, H, told me today that she is also pregnant. Our kids will be like twins, she said. We can have playdates, I said. How wonderful. She will be an incredible mother. So happy for her, even though she appears to be a Fertile Myrtle (and we hate Fertile Myrtles).

63

Sea Monkey

Okay so I know that at five weeks my 'baby' is actually more like an embryo, or maybe a foetus, but I am loving watching him grow. I have one of those apps on my phone that tells you that your little one is as big as a poppyseed, then a grapefruit, then a watermelon (we are still at 'pea' stage), and tells you what is developing and shows you how it looks, from sea monkey to fish to reptile to alien (we are still at sea monkey). I whip my phone out at inappropriate moments and show people my little pea-sized sea monkey.

Stinging Nipples

No, this is not the name of a new rock band. It's an entirely unexpected symptom of pregnancy.

In The Womb

Mike and I watched the documentary called 'In The Womb' — It's about (spoiler alert) the development of babies in utero. Amazing! Here I thought with my little file from when I was 8 years old that I knew everything, courtesy of 1987 Fair Lady magazines and my mother's copy of 'Everywoman'.

It made me feel a bit breathless at times, the way so many things can go wrong, or not happen when they should. No wonder this having babies business is so fraught with peril. The most nail-biting moment is right in the beginning when the cells that form the heart are doing their thing and they make this tiny, tiny little chamber (and you think: Look, guys, this is *never* going to work) and then you're watching that still, silent pocket, holding your breath, and something, some pulse, some invisible lightning bolt from heaven hits it and the little heart begins to gallop along. Incredible. Awe-inspiring.

Absolutely fucking terrifying.

...

I have, after reading Gretchen Rubin's book, 'The Happiness Project,' come up with my own personal commandments. Like life, it's a work in progress.

1. Keep It Simple

2. Keep a sense of humour

3. 80/20 rule

4. Have less, do more, love more

5. Choose not to take things personally

6. Be generous

7. Be selfish

8. Keep walking

9. Cut yourself some slack

10. Always have a project to work on

11. Always be in the middle of a great book

12. Identify Perfect Moments

13. Write

14. Grow things

15. Know that magic happens

THE TRIPS ARE KICKING

Very tired lately and finding it impossible to concentrate. I find the days are way too long, but still don't have enough hours in them to get everything done. Didn't sleep well last night: thirsty, hungry, itchy.

A lot of twinging down there so I tell Mike that the trips are kicking.

Bernadette came over for tea and to give us plant-cuttings from Dugmore street in Port Elizabeth (Mike's gran is moving out of the big family house they have lived in for decades. It was just her rattling around in there after Jack died.) It was touching, to be able to keep some of Dugmore street in our garden. I planted them with extra compost. We went for an evening walk and made dinner together. So happy.

Tree Triplets

Lovely day at the nursery buying trees for the garden. Nausea set off by the disgusting car air freshener that I've never noticed before. I had to hang out the window like a labrador. We bought fruiting olive trees, Virginia Creeper, and three Giant Pock Ironwoods. I, for a change, didn't want to get my hands dirty, but I cheered Mike on as he dug huge holes for the Ironwoods and planted them, three in a row. They look wonderful. Our tree triplets!

We took our first 'belly pics' — first in skimpy undies and then a more PC version. Feeling very happy, hungry and fat. Swollen tummy and boobs. Eating loads despite feeling huge. Been walking every day and doing gentle yoga afterwards. Battling to focus on work or writing — just want to spend all day reading pregnancy books, napping and eating.

Eating for Four

Mike and I met Msibi for home-made ice cream at

Trieste in Greenside. We were celebrating the Big Fat Positive. Msibi gave me loads of (orange! clever friend) body butter, most likely to stave off the stretch marks I am dying to get. Satsuma.

The ice cream was delicious. My favourite was rose-petal flavour, although it did taste a bit like Lux soap smells. The coconut was also delicious. I always order the five-scoop bowl, so that I get to taste as many flavours as possible. There were, of course, the requisite jokes, that I am now eating for four, with the triplets on board.

ALL-DAY-SICKNESS

I have started to get morning sickness. It's revolting. I love it. It feels as though your brain is queasy. Vomit is never far away. The idea of food is disgusting but the only way to feel better is to eat, like a Möbius ribbon of not-yet-chundered-up-food. If you even think about vomming, saliva gushes into your mouth until you look at the ceiling and force yourself to picture calming scenes: ocean-polished glass, cold pebbles, clear seas.

Being pregnant is like having one long, vicious hangover. Constant nausea, exhaustion, all-over-body-ache, the gnawing need for food that you don't want to eat. It's easy to say no to booze when your body is wrapped up in this woozy fug; and, despite not drinking a drop of alcohol, you wake up every morning with the hangover you went to bed with the night before. The Neverending Hangover. Part I, II, II, IV, V, ad infinitum.

It's revolting but I love it because every twinge in my stomach, every rush of nausea confirms that I am still pregnant. The heavy feeling in my uterus could be the beginning of a period, the stinging nipples come and go, but the sickness is loyal and stays with me all day.

FINE

We are going for our first scan tomorrow. I am so glad the wait is over, and so nervous. On the one hand I wake up every morning with this quiet happy confidence that I am pregnant, really pregnant. On the other hand I feel: How can I be this lucky? Something is bound to be wrong. I haven't had this bitter edge before; I used to think of myself as fortunate. The cynicism is a gift, a leftover, a pain-stain from infertility. Everyone is rallying around us in their respective emails. They're all saying: 'It will be FINE!'

Text from Mike: Very excited for our first scan. Wow it's exciting.

POST OFFICE MISCARRIAGE

I got the fright of my life today, standing in the queue at the local post office. I hate that dismal, depressing room with its out-of-date sun-bleached posters and dirty cream-coloured walls. When I'm in there I always have the urge to paint the place. Or if they can't afford a coat of paint, couldn't they at least wash the grubby walls? Polish the wood? The notices stuck to the smeared glass partitions with old Prestik shout at you in uppercase Comic Sans, insulting you with bad grammar and nonsensical clauses. The people are nice, and that makes it worse. I feel sorry for them having to face this dreary-as-shit place every day with its crumbling ceiling boards and broken air conditioner.

Yesterday I felt my shoulder twinge. It was nothing, I told myself. It was nothing it was nothing it was nothing. Just a memory of pain. Or perhaps the pregnancy hormones are irritating it a bit. It's not impossible.

I was standing there, waiting my turn, parcel collection slips in hand, trying not to tap my foot, when it happened. I had had an achy, full-feeling uterus all morning and as I stood there staring at a picture of an envelope flying around the world I felt this sudden warm gush out of my baby canon.

No, no no no no no, I thought, please God no. Not a miscarriage. Not here, not now, not ever. Perhaps someone else would have called their doctor, or driven straight to hospital, but I thought, sadly: if it has happened, it has happened. There is no un-miscarrying. There is no re-carrying. I left, walked slowly to the car, grateful that I had parked so close, and that I was wearing a dark pair of jeans. When I peeled them off at home I expected them to be slimy with blood, but there was no red, just what looked like water. Is it possible, I wondered, that my water had broken so early in the pregnancy? Was there even 'water' to break? I guessed there would be, a little bit. Everything else seemed fine: no cramping, nothing else out of the ordinary. I asked the girls on the forum what it could be. The general consensus was that it was just a side effect from the progesterone pessaries, and that I should get used to it, because when you are pregnant you are almost always wet down there. Good for spontaneous sex, not so good for your state of mind when you're standing in a dingy post office. Tomorrow's scan couldn't come any sooner.

64

A Heartbeat

So very, very lucky. It looks like this baby IS a survivor. We had our first scan today with dear doctor G (how I love that man) and there the baby was, in black and white, a perfect little sea monkey. The most beautiful sea monkey I have ever seen. The moment before the scan was the most anxious I have ever been in my life. It was like the opposite of dying — a wash of yellow adrenaline as I saw my infertility flash before my eyes — and then it all fell away as we focused on the screen that came to life before us: a galaxy of white noise and stars, and in the centre a small — the smallest — human, singular, with A HEARTBEAT. Brave little thing, hammering away! It sounded like a galloping horse. No, not an ordinary horse. More magical than that: a galloping unicorn. The girls on the forum had told me it would be the best sound I have ever heard, and they were right. I was ready to weep, from the relief, from the joy, but all I managed were a few lone-wolf tears. I was, in fact, too happy to cry.

We went to Fournos afterwards for lunch, a mini-celebration. I caught my reflection in a mirror and didn't recognise the disgustingly cheerful woman glowing back at me.

I took a video of the ultrasound on my phone to show everyone in the Mike Jnr Fan Club. I must have watched it a hundred times today.

65

Grooving and Sparring

Had our second (10-week) scan today. Tiny pea has grown so much (35mm) and was dancing for us. It's like he knew he had an audience. He was bopping and moonwalking like a mini version of Michael Jackson. We were all laughing. It was a perfect moment. Later he floated upside-down and hung from the top of his cave like a bat. I thought: If he ever has a brother we can call him 'Robin'. He also showed us his boxing moves (my dad would be so proud) and played with his thumbs. He's the size of an olive, and he has thumbs! It was so wonderful, so powerful. I thought I would cry but my smile was so wide my tear-ducts didn't stand a chance.

Back in his office afterwards, Dr G said: 'Well done, Lawrence cubed!' (his first name is Lawrence).

He's referred us to a high-risk obstetrician. All IVF pregnancies, no matter how healthy they look, are considered 'high-risk,' but apart from that, he has a concern.

He said that when they did the embryo transfers it was uncommonly easy to thread the catheter through my cervix, which leads him to suspect that it is incompetent. (I know! How rude! My poor cervix is still smarting.) It's not a big deal at all, according to Dr G, if you recognise it in time. We can just 'stitch it up'. So, we have a complication. It's not the end of the world. I can count my lucky stars that I am in such good hands. Losing a healthy baby after Everything doesn't bear thinking about.

I know about cervical stitches from the forum, but also because my mom lost her second pregnancy to her incompetent cervix (sorry, mom's cervix! I don't mean to hurt your feelings. I actually have great regard for you).

Dr G told us that after the surgeries I have had on my uterus, natural birth is no longer an option. It has been 'compromised' and may, in the final stage of labour, 'blow its top'.

Ha! Funny. Funny enough to make me laugh in his office, but I do need to mini-mourn the idea I've always had of having a natural birth. More specifically, a beautiful water birth. Some women dream of their wedding day (pssh!) — I used to fantasise about giving birth. I'm the kind of person who watches YouTube videos of other people giving birth. I find it fascinating. I'm sure I was a midwife/doula in a previous life.

My Swiss host-mother used to tell me that giving birth felt so close to death and then there is this new life that you have created and it's the most intense experience ever.

I thought the idea of having to have a C-section would upset me more than it has. I guess I have a better perspective now — I know that the only thing that matters is having a healthy baby. I'm also not the same naïve hippie I was in the beginning of this journey, eschewing any kind of surgery as 'too invasive'. Now I'm just happy (overjoyed) that there is an ACTUAL BABY to be talking about.

So we have a compromised uterus and an incompetent cervix. No one said this was going to be easy.

Saying goodbye to Dr G was bittersweet.

66

12 WEEKS

WE MADE IT TO 12 WEEKS. Mike Jnr is alive and kicking. We are officially in the second trimester. Our new doc, the high-risk obstetrician, did a FAS (foetal anomaly scan) and gave us the thumbs up. He asked if we wanted to test for Downs, etc., but we said no. The baby was bouncing around in his little black bubble. It was so lovely to see him. I wish we could have a scan every day. Oh, how I love him already. It makes me clench my jaw when I think of it.

Pregnant with a healthy baby. Only now do I realise how stressful the first trimester was. Yes, I was walking on air most of the time, waking up — still pregnant — was like a gift in my palm every morning. But reaching 12 weeks has magnified that feeling. Now there is a very high chance that I will actually have a living, breathing, yelling, crying, sleeping baby in six months' time. Seems too good to be true. I can't believe my luck. The mind boggles.

RVR (the new doc) agrees that I need a cervical stitch, and we're doing it next week. I am happy to get it done — I would agree to absolutely anything that would mean I could keep this baby baking for as long as possible. It's a really simple procedure, he said. Unfortunately it requires general anaesthetic, which I don't like the idea of, but he says that the baby will just have a nice sleep, no side-effects, and I am not to worry. It doesn't make sense to think about it really, as I know that without the stitch I will lose the pregnancy. In that case, what's a little anaesthetic between friends? It's not like I'm not used to it. It will be the fifth time I will go under in less than two years.

We like RVR. He gives the impression that he really knows what he is doing. He makes me feel safe.

He said I should try not to put on more than 10kg during the pregnancy. That will be difficult seeing as I've already put on 4kg and around 23 grams of that is Baby. How are you supposed to not put on weight when you have to nosh constantly to keep the nausea at bay? Some people say that pregnant women use their pregnancy as an excuse to overeat. Well, I'd like to high-five those people in the face. It's not like I sit in the front of the TV and eat doughnuts. Okay, sometimes I do, but my point is that not putting on pregnancy weight is a lot more difficult than you'd think, especially when you've cut out running and yoga to make sure the baby sticks.

My favourite part of the day is 4pm when I go for a long walk. I plug in my music and walk to Zoo Lake and back. It's 8km and takes me around an hour. I spend the time day-dreaming of my baby.

The biggest news, apart from getting through the first trimester, is that RVR saw something on the scan and asked if we'd like to know the gender of the baby. We said, we already knew. It's a boy! And he said, yes, you're right.

IT'S A BOY! I'm going to have a baby boy. I'm going to have a son.

James

Mike and I went out for dinner to celebrate hitting the all-important 12-week mark. We're basking in our mutual optimism for the future and, in such a happy space, everything tasted amazing. I'm so over-the-top cheerful that I don't even miss drinking wine, which I previously wouldn't have believed possible.

Dr RVR said that a lot of the pregnancy 'rules' are bullshit. As long as you're not drinking, drugging or smoking you don't need to cut anything else out. Sushi? I asked. He said he wouldn't like to the be the one telling an entire country of pregnant Japanese women not to eat sushi. Tuna? I asked, having heard of the high mercury level in the fish. Pssh! He says. You breathe in more mercury in one breath down in a parking basement than you could ingest from eating a ton of tinned tuna.

Note to self: No more parking in basements. For a high-risk doctor, he seems pretty easy-going.

We decided on Mike Jnr's real name years ago, as well as his imaginary sister's, but we talked about it more tonight. We will call him James. I love the sound of the word, its simplicity. I love that it starts with a J, like mine does, that it is common but not too common. Something about it feels right, as if I somehow know deep down that I WILL have a son named James. As if I have been there and seen it for myself. James, I say out loud, James.

Sitting at the restaurant with Mike, talking about our little olive and baby names instead of turkey basting and painkillers and hormone shots. Looking forward to the future with bright eyes instead of the fear and anxiety the pain used to bring, I wonder if I have found the meaning in my suffering. This amped-up joy, this almost overwhelming sense of love I feel: would I have felt like this if I had been a Fertile Myrtle? If I had fallen pregnant as soon as Mike had 'hung his underwear on the line'? I know that infertility has made me a better person, hopefully it's made me a better friend, and it will most certainly make me a better parent. But is this enough? It doesn't seem proportionate. Perhaps it will become clearer in time.

...

I was chatting to Mandie about how much I love my pain specialist, Dr Finegan. I think that pain management was a very important part in the success of the third IVF. I was saying how I'd like to do something nice for her. Bake her a cake, maybe. Send her flowers. Mandie suggested sending a singing telegram, which made me think: what would they sing? I started putting a few words down and it became a really silly poem. I wish I could draw like Quentin Blake — then I'd illustrate it like a children's book and give it to her.

A (Silly) Ode to Dr Finegan

There was a time I was in bitterbright pain

My shoulder was burning, it near drove me insane.

Diaphragmatic endometriosis was the bane of my life

I wanted to cut off my arm with a knife.

I spent days and nights on couches, crying

Sometimes I felt like I was dead-and-or-dying.

Hot water bottles, tablets, they didn't help a lick

I needed something stronger to really do the trick.

A doctor I met referred me to you

See a pain specialist, he said, it's the only thing to do

He saw how the pills I was on, hurt my tummy

He said, listen here, go see Dr Finegan, dummy!

She'll give you some chronic pain medication

It'll be like your shoulder upped and went on vacation

The Underachieving Ovary

There's no point in hurting as much as you do

Go see her, and soon, you'll feel good as new.

Dr Finegan, lovely lady, pain specialist, esquire

Saw that my situation was terrible and dire

She didn't hesitate, she didn't spin any yarns

She wrote me a prescription as long as my arm.

A script of painkillers! Rainbow ice cream!

Marshmallow pillows! Candyfloss dreams!

Anti-inflammatories! Analgesic cocktails galore!

At last my body could rest, my shoulder wasn't sore!

Dear doctor Finegan

You're in my thoughts again-again

You verily, honestly, changed my life

You took away my pain (you took away the knife).

67

In Stitches

Holy Fucking Shitballs that stitch hurt like a mothertrucker. My slacker of a cervix had a major problem with being reigned in, and threw a temper tantrum. Calling them 'cramps' would be a vast understatement. Describing them as 'uncomfortable' would be like calling the 2004 Tsunami 'a big wave'. The elastic they use is like the strip you find in your *broeks* and they thread it into your muscle good and proper so that there is no way it can come out under the pressure of a baby trying to make an early exit. They cinch it shut like a money bag. A MacDonald's Cerclage is the medical term. You get other kinds of cervical stitches, but my doc is a MacDonald's fan.

Before they knocked me out in the OR I made sure that everyone knew that this pregnancy had been a long time coming and was (is) the most important thing in the world to me. I looked them all in the eyes and told them.

When I woke up, the first thing I asked the nurse

was if my baby was okay, and when she said a loud, assuring YES I started bawling (I sense that there is to be a fair amount of outright weeping over the next few months). I was so relieved. I know it wasn't a risky procedure but I had obviously been a lot more anxious about it than I had realised. Then the anaesthetic started wearing off and all I was allowed to take was paracetamol. I looked at the two white tabs and then at the nurse as if to say: You're kidding, right? There is an angry rhinoceros stomping on my uterus and you give me fucking paracetamol? I swallowed them, but knew that if I had stuck them in my ear or chucked them out of the window they would have had the same effect. Don't get me wrong, I don't want to drug my baby, but Holy Moses it was sore. The nurse, seeing my 'discomfort,' pulled out her own version of 'the big guns' and gave me a latex glove and an anti-inflammatory suppository in a plastic cup. My usual reaction to the offer of a suppository would be a red-faced 'No thanks!' a little louder than necessary (because arbitrary people go around offering me suppositories all the time) but on this occasion the supp was gone before the nurse even turned around, leaving the glove in the bin and an empty spinning cup on my bedside table. My expert first-time suppository dexterity surprised even me.

I wanted to keep the cramping under control obviously because it was painful, but mostly because I was worried about what it was doing to Mike Jnr. He is still so tiny (although he has graduated from olive to sugar plum) and the intensity of the squeezing couldn't have been good; or maybe I am just overprotective (i.e. paranoid) and overreacting. I told Pin afterwards that the cramping was scary and she said: He'll be fine! He's so cosy. Just think about them as nice big hugs.

...

I don't know what anaesthetic they used on me yesterday but I feel like I've been hit by an especially large truck. Holy Moses! Did I do an Iron Man yesterday without knowing it? Full body stiffness, blinding headache. I can't even look at my screen, never mind work. Lovely Mike is packing all my orders to be dispatched. If it sounds like I'm complaining, I am, but really, I'm not. It feels good knowing that baba is stitched in nice and snugly.

...

We saw the Kings of Leon last night. It was weird going to a concert pregnant (and sober). It's like you can focus on the music more, but the high emotion that usually comes with the combination of the flat beer and the performance is missing. I took it easy, didn't dance too much. I think that the sugar plum enjoyed it (although I think he actually may be a lime, by now).

We ate King Cones. They were good. Life is good.

Also: we are allowed to have sex again! After a very long three months of holy abstinence. The only problem is: condoms. In the most ironic twist of ironic twists everywhere since the beginning of time, my infertile and pregnant self has to make use of rubbers. Ha ha, universe, I thought to myself, Ha ha. Why don't I just start taking the pill, while I'm at it. Throw in a cap, why don't you, and an IUD.

Because of the stitch, we have to be super cautious.

I am on a truckload of antibiotics for the rest of the pregnancy and, apart from the condoms, we are also not allowed to try any 'funny stuff.' I was dying to ask Dr RVR what exactly, in his mind, qualifies as 'funny stuff.' Medical clowns? B.A. Baracas impersonations? Dogs running into sliding doors? I clamped my mouth shut. 'No funny stuff' I typed into my phone, and gave Mike the beady eye.

. . .

Ach, this pregnancy. I DO love it, but it's making me so sick. The girls on the forum always feel bad about complaining about pregnancy symptoms (there is a special 'room' for us preggos that IFers enter at their own peril) because it was all they wanted for years and now that they have it they don't dare complain, even if their back/morning sickness/feet are killing them. I say: bullshit! Revel in the symptoms. Moan all you like! You have worked harder for the nausea/swollen ankles than most living people. You've had enough of a hard time. Complain all you like.

But, secretly, I feel the guilt, too. How can I, in good conscience, after everything, groan about anything? Well, I can't, not in polite company anyway, and not to the friends and family who agonised with me over my infertility. But I can write it down in this labrador-loyal journal. So here goes:

I feel pukey and exhausted ALL THE TIME and I have broken out in an awful case of eczema all over my legs and hips that keeps me awake at night. It's as itchy as Hades. When I do fall asleep I get vicious calf cramps that make me jump awake. My back aches constantly, even in bed. Food revolts me. Eating saves me. But there are only very specific things I can eat, which change daily and with vehemence.

...

Gill is in ICU again. They had to operate, again: that laparotomy that I was so afraid of, when they gut you like a fish. She has now had two in as many years. The fright still hasn't left my Dad's face. I gave him a long hug. You okay, Captain? I asked. He nodded. Pretended to be cross with Gill for scaring him.

The first time it happened they were out in the bush in the middle of nowhere. They had to be evacuated, Gill given the emergency, life-saving surgery. At least this time they were home when it happened. I hated seeing her look so ill. Usually so vibrant, she cut a desperate figure lying on those starched sheets, a hundred stitches richer.

We talked about how plump I was looking, how healthy. When you get out of here we'll need to fatten you up too, I thought.

A couple of months ago Dad gave Denton and I a copy of his will. He has diabetes. You wouldn't guess it by looking at him: ruddy cheeked and relaxed from his early retirement and years spent travelling Southern Africa. He has a book listing 101 pubs to visit in SA and he takes it very seriously. He gets the bartender to sign the relevant pages and shows the book to us when we visit, telling us the story behind each one. I've told him that we need to write a follow-up together, with his vignettes. He's happy with his complimentary T-shirts and beer mugs.

Recently he met a parrot on one of his watering hole sojourns who likes to drink tomato cocktails. You would buy him a can from the bar and the bird would thank you, open the tin himself, and chug back a Virgin Mary. Gold! I tell him. You can't make this stuff up.

You need to get well soon, I told Gill. You haven't finished visiting all the pubs in that book. My Dad, emotional, puffs up: You tell her, Neets.

...

Chris took us to Dullstroom and then Leadwood Lodge for a mini-holiday, along with Simon. Luxury! We ate strawberries and cream in the middle of the bush and saw all the big 5 in one game drive. Chris had a word with the ranger for driving too fast — he explained that we had some special cargo on board.

68

WHO'S MY LITTLE RUTABAGA?

16 WEEKS

It seems we have another complication. A serious one. I'm trying not to worry.

We had our 16-week scan today and RVR says that I have a severe case of placenta praevia. He noticed it in the previous scan — but often the placenta moves up with the uterus as it expands — but he can now see that this one is here to stay. Praevia is when the placenta covers, or partially covers, the cervix (the baby's exit gate). You get four grades of severity and, yes, you guessed it, we have grade four, AKA complete praevia, which means that the placenta covers the entire cervix. RVR said that if there was a grade five, we would have it. In the old days the mother had no chance of surviving childbirth, even if she had a C-section. I only Googled enough to learn about the basics. I stopped when I came across placenta accreta, which happens in 5-10% of praevia cases. It is when the placental tissue grows too deeply into the womb, attaching to the muscle layer, and may result in life-threatening haemorrhaging and a hysterectomy. Now I'm not always on speaking terms with my uterus, but I would be devastated to lose it. Usually I would read all the gory details about accreta and scare the shitkittens out of myself, but now I can't stress about it. I have Mike Jnr to think about. I stopped when I came across this list. Usually I really like lists. This one, not so much.

Some of the complications of placenta praevia include:

- Major haemorrhage (bleeding) for the mother
- Shock from loss of blood
- Foetal distress from lack of oxygen
- Premature labour or delivery
- Health risks to the baby, if born prematurely
- Emergency caesarean delivery
- Hysterectomy, if the placenta fails to come away from the uterine lining
- Blood loss for the baby
- Death.

I like how they just throw that last one in there like that. Thanks WebMD.

. . .

Gold-hearted Simon gave us a gift: a 4D scan that he'd bought on a special offer. The clinic was in the South so my mom came with us and we went to Gino's afterwards for dinner. Mike Jnr was shy in the beginning, but quickly warmed up to us and played a bit, and kept putting his hand in his mouth and on his chin, as if he was having a good think. He looks very much like an alien, but we love him anyway. Very skinny, with pronounced rib- and cheekbones. A skinny baby alien, what's not to love?

Pin has been so kind, letting us borrow her baby stuff. So special. And our friends keep giving us gifts. Teddies, blankets, finger puppets! A customer of mine — who I have never met — made two beautiful quilts for us. I am continually amazed by the generosity that surrounds us. So very grateful that it is difficult to put into words. It's as if the world has turned (back) into a benevolent place.

LIFE OR DEATH

They started bashing down walls today. I didn't realise they would start so soon. I was running around digging up plants, to rescue them. The page in 'What To Expect When You're Expecting' was haunting me as I plunged my hands into the soil, the one that says if you have cats you're not to garden when pregnant because of toxoplasmosis. Squatting there elbow-deep in mud, Alex rubbing up against me, it occurred to me that we would be renovating for most of the pregnancy.

Only an insane person would agree to renovate while pregnant. I obviously didn't truly believe it would happen. Any pregnancy guide will tell you that while you are preparing for the birth you should make sure any small DIY jobs, like replacing lightbulbs, are done well in advance of bringing baby home. Fuck, I thought, as our (only) bathroom wall came crashing down.

. . .

Terrible news. H just let me know that they lost the baby. They went for their 12-week scan today and there was no heartbeat. Devastating! She had to go in for a D&C. Terrible, absolutely terrible. I hope that she and her husband heal soon. Can you ever truly get over losing a child? My heart aches for them. I can't help feeling that it should have been me.

. . .

Lying awake at night, considering this: how doctors have had a life or death influence over me without me even knowing it, before now. If my mother had been with a high-risk obstetrician during her second pregnancy, she wouldn't have lost her second son, Spencer, and I would never have been conceived. I wouldn't have lived.

And in my own life: if I had been living a hundred years ago, pre-IVF, I wouldn't have been able to get pregnant. Without painkillers and doctors with a clue, my shoulder would have landed me on a fiery stake, or in the loony bin, like Hilary Mantel, or I would have taken my own life. And if by some miracle I had managed to conceive before the endo set in (perhaps because I would have married at 16), I would have died in childbirth. No one survived placenta praevia in those days.

Perhaps 100 years ago infertility would have killed me.

Or my heart-shaped uterus would have stopped me

from conceiving, and in doing so, save me from the praevia.

Perhaps 100 years ago my infertility would have saved my life.

18 WEEKS

One of Chris's friend's is very good at saying exactly the wrong thing. I forgive her because A) She clearly doesn't have a clue how barbed her comments are. I don't think she means any harm. She's also B) Kind of dating Chris so dinners out would be awkward if I wasn't talking to her.

We had a braai at Chris's house today and while we were getting drinks in the kitchen she comes up to me and pokes me in the stomach. 'Wow!' she says in her weird accent. 'You've REALLY put on weight, haven't you?'

'I'm pregnant!' I say, pulling in my tummy.

'Yes,' she says, 'I know, but look at this!' she says, jiggling my love handles. She is fascinated. 'Isn't it incredible,' she marvels, 'how all the weight settles in this area.'

'Yes,' I say, downing my rock shandy before I give into the temptation to pour it down her irritatingly thin body. I've decided I don't like her figure: she's too skinny. Sis! I say to myself. Like a stick figure, but a dry, grey one, like driftwood on a desert beach.

Later, once I have forgiven her, the conversation

wheels around to cosmetic surgery, and then Botox. She says everyone is doing it now. I thought that by 'everyone' she meant people her age, but either way I didn't care enough to argue.

'Just a bit of Botox here, some filler there,' she says. She looks straight at me: 'You'll be going for that kind of thing soon.'

...

All I want to eat is Marmite and cheddar. Mike says that if I keep eating like this I'm going to give birth to a Marmite and cheese sandwich. I crave orange juice, the more acidic the better. Fruit has never tasted better. Minneolas! Oh my, Minneolas. Where have you been all my life? I crave vinegar and protein. I can't stand the sight of salad or any fresh vegetables. I've realised that I'm not even getting half the protein I'm supposed to be getting, so the house is no longer a vegetarian abode. There is always a packet of quickly-diminishing biltong in the fridge. I count the grams of protein like a bodybuilder. I need 75g a day. I eat a lot of eggs. Soon I'll be able to bench-press my own body weight in yellow cheese.

20 WEEKS

I have a bump! I have a proper pregnant belly. It kind of popped out. Now people I see don't have to panic that I've become fat overnight. They don't have to walk on that uncomfortable ledge of 'When are you due?' vs. 'Whoah! Who ate all the pies?'

Sleeping is starting to get uncomfortable. When I turn over all my organs have to rearrange themselves to get comfy again. Strangest sensation.

I've also started to feel movement. Not the 'butterflies' or 'popcorn popping' I've heard about, but a deep, achy slow movement, like you get after eating a burger from a trailer outside a nightclub at 3am.

...

I finished the first draft of my new novel, 'Why You Were Taken', and I'm happy with it. It needs some re-working but essentially I like the story and I enjoyed writing it. Once I finish the third draft I'll start submitting it to publishers. I still think you can tell that I wrote it while I was in the blue haze. Hopefully I'll be able to take out the emotional distance in the rewrite.

...

The girls on the forum were talking about if they will tell their children about being IVF babies or not. I say, of course! Not only does it make the Birds & Bees talk easier (So Mommy and Daddy went to the doctor and he put a baby in Mommy's tummy) but when they start to understand it, they will realise that not only were they wanted, they were really, REALLY wanted. R250,000 worth of Wanted (and just so that you know, kiddo, we'll be docking your pocket money until you've paid us back in full, with interest. Best you become a child star or similar. We'll let you off until you have some kind of neck control, but after that you'll need to pull your weight. All 2kg of it). In the meantime we'll dress you in a onesie that says: 'I am the reason Mom can't have nice things.'

Minty Sensations

Mike and I were standing in a pharmacy, looking at the different condoms on offer. We are not experienced condom-buyers and both hate the things but needs must. We marvelled at the selection available. Like out-of-town hicks stumbling into a New York coffee bar, the menu flummoxed us. I imagined a condom-barista appearing: *Double-length, half-latex, ultra-thin, hold the lube?* he would suggest. We would swallow our questions and nod. *Would you like a complimentary biscotti with that?*

What about these, I said, holding up a box of rubbers with what looked like an oiled mechanic on the packaging. Mike was wearing his poker face. Maybe mechanics aren't his thing.

These? I said, tapping a box of Ribbed & Studded.

These? Looking at a packet of Minty Sensations. Who knew you could get mint-flavoured condoms? I certainly didn't. I thought that they should be in the toothpaste aisle, or with the chewing gum at the till.

Another couple approached — seasoned vets, compared to us, despite their tender age — and grabbed what I guessed was their usual. Their only hesitation was when they saw my 5-month baby bump jutting out in front of me. They seemed genuinely puzzled. I could sense they wanted to tell us that it was too late for condoms, but decided to mind their own Ribbed & Studdeds.

I wanted to call out after them: They don't always work, you know! and pat my bulge, as a joke. Instead we just grabbed the same ones they had and beat a hasty retreat. We should have bought more, I thought, when we got to the cashier and faced another non-plussed frown. I didn't know how many more blushing sessions I can stand.

21 WEEKS

I felt the baby move for the first time. A high tap-tap-tapping in my tummy. Amazing! Hello baba, I say to my bump. Hello my baba.

22 WEEKS

Mike felt the baby kick for the first time! We were at Dad and Gill's for Xmas eve and I felt him move so Mike put his hand on my bump and the little sausage kicked! Then everyone had a turn to feel and we all stood around smiling at each other like dorks. Next Xmas we will have a little 8-month-old baby. He'll be eating solids already, maybe even crawling. Unbelievable.

23 WEEKS

I am already getting Braxton Hicks contractions. They scare the hell out of me. I got them so badly the other day when I was walking to the *spruit* with Mike that we had to turn back. They are 'fake' mini contractions, your uterus supposedly practising for the real thing, but they are alarming when they are intense enough to double you over at five-and-a-bit months pregnant. Okay 'uterus,' I want to say. I get it. You fucked up the whole 'falling pregnant' thing 26 cycles in a row and now that you're hosting a mango you feel the need to overcompensate. Well, don't! Your contraction services are not needed, now, or ever. Just keep that baby baking. That's all you have to do. Don't fuck it up!

WHO'S MY LITTLE RUTABAGA?

Mike Jnr is now, according to my app, as big as a rutabaga. WTF is a rutabaga? I had to Google it. It looks like a golden beetroot. Now I can't stop saying it, in a bad American accent. Roo-da-bay-gah, I say, patting my bump. Roo-da-bay-gah. Who's my little roodabaygah? I scrolled on a few weeks and saw that at 32 weeks he'll be as big as a jicama. Again, what? A jicama, from what I can see, is a superbly ugly potato. And then 33 weeks is even better: a durian! Turns out that a durian is the 'King of Fruits' in Asia, AKA the Stink Fruit. I remember seeing them in Thailand. I can't wait to call him my little Stink Fruit.

. . .

Today I am officially a published author. 'The Memory of Water' is on the shelves. (Or, rather, off the shelves — my friends and Mom, Dad and Chris keep buying up all my stock!) Amazing Mandie designed the cover and it's beautiful. It is my baby, in a way. I am lucky enough that — unlike Mantel — I will have a baby and a book, rather than books instead of babies. My next book is almost finished. I have to get it done before Mike Junior arrives. Best get cracking.

69

PLEASE KEEP BAKING, BABY

24 WEEKS

24-week scan today and all is good with baba. The placenta is still a problem, though. RVR expects me to start bleeding at any time and says that we will roll with the punches when I do. The size of the baby needs to be weighed up against the amount of blood loss I'll experience and there is nothing we can do about it now except take steroid shots. The steroids will speed up the maturation of the baby's lungs (lungs are last to finish developing in utero) so that even if we are forced to do an emergency c-section really early on he will have a better chance of thriving. It's scary, thinking he'll be premature.

Every day that I don't bleed I thank my lucky stars. Every day that the praevia doesn't affect this pregnancy is a day that James can grow and put on weight, and his lungs can develop. I picture him turning from a banana into a brinjal, into a coconut, which makes me thirsty for a Piña

341

Colada. Or, rather, a Piña un-Colada. We're at 25 weeks today. Please keep baking, baby.

70

IT ONLY TAKES ONE, AND OTHER STORIES

I would like to write a non-fiction book about couples beating infertility. There are so many 'miracle' stories on the forum, I'd love to write about them. There was this one girl, I'll call her Want2BMum (because they always have names like that on FC. You're never getting advice from a Betty or a Barbara, but a Been_Too_Long). Want2BMum went through the usual horrible rigmarole of Infertility for Dummies, the whole rude introduction of bad eggs, bad sperm, or a bad combination of both. She had to do IVF if she wanted a chance to conceive. The stimming didn't go very well, the retrieval was worse, and the result was that she only had one egg to work with. One egg! Absolutely devastating. I think I may have jumped off a cliff. But the egg was successfully fertilised and then they had one embryo, which was at least something. She couldn't believe how badly it had gone and had a stomp around the forum. We all rallied round her, sympathised with her, told her that 'It only takes one!' although I'm sure that none of us really believed she had a chance. The important thing was that she believed that she had a chance. We could deal with the actual result later, after the two-week wait. It only takes one, she kept telling herself, it only takes one. And yes, she got her Big Fat Positive.

There are lots of other stories to be told. Some tragic, most life-affirming. Some are just good stories. One of my cycle buddies (the women who do IVF in the same month as you and you track each others' progress) was busy with a cycle using a surrogate. I think it was their third or fourth attempt at IVF. Their surro got pregnant (yay!) and then a month later my cycle buddy was pregnant too, without any treatment. Basically, she's having twins. Except she'll have a couple of months to practise changing nappies on the one baby before the other one comes along. It gives the saying 'my brother from another mother' a whole new meaning.

...

I was wondering if maybe the purpose of the pain was to push us into action. A cruel catalyst. Neither of us wanted to pursue fertility treatments initially, but the pain gave me little option. It held us hostage. It was get pregnant or die.

If it hadn't pushed us so hard, we probably would still be waiting (not-so-patiently) here, after three years, and I'd still have a heart-shaped uterus and twisted tubes. By the time we finally decided to try treatment it would have been too late. There would to too much damage done by the endo, and not an egg to be seen.

Perhaps the pain — and I really hate to admit this

— was exactly what we needed in order to conceive.

I guess that you can peel the onion of destiny in many ways. In this layer of onion the pain compelled me to do whatever it took to realise my dream, and the pain takes on a heroic glow. Peel one more layer, though, and the endo doesn't exist at all, and the pain is back to being a complete bastard that no one needs in order to get pregnant. You need to decide on an angle. Think of the tabloid headline possibilities, from: 'The Pain That Almost Ruined My Life' to 'Shoulder Pain Saved My Fertility Dream'. The bones of the story remain the same, it's how you tell it that changes everything.

...

Chris has had bad news from his oncologist. We're looking at a year now, maybe two. I am devastated. He is such a big, generous presence in our lives. Always so supportive with his thoughtful, rational discourse and his (albeit distant) affection. Always having us over for hamburger braais and teaching us about GDP while we teach him about Twitter and Facebook.

Sometimes he 'pops in' unannounced with a cappuccino and a croissant for me. As benevolent as the gesture is, I used to find it mildly irritating: constantly under the gun to finish my work, needing to get invoices processed and parcels dispatched, not in the mood (or dressed) for unexpected visitors (certainly not when I was in pain or trying to see through the blue haze of the Trepiline). He'd just want a 'quick chat' (there's no such thing as a free cappuccino) — while I sat there watching the clock tick. I am ashamed now of my lack of graciousness.

The truth is that he helped us to conceive. He talked me down from the moral high-horse of IVF costs, he listened to our every Big Fat Negative disappointment. He made invaluable cash injections into the Mike Jnr slush fund. Now I am pregnant with his first grandson and he won't live to see him grow up. I find this knowledge savagely sad. I've been crying all day.

OH, MY ACHING CERVIX

25 WEEKS

Before TTCing I had no idea where the cervix actually was. Now I could draw a map. Now we're on a first-name basis. I talk to her, tell her she's doing a good job despite the rocky start with the whole 'incompetency' issue. I know that feelings had been hurt. Assure her that she is not, as she suspects, up for retrenchment.

Just one trimester to go.

71

DEMENTED GAME OF MUSICAL CHAIRS

It doesn't look like the builders will be done in time. We keep moving our bed around the house like a demented game of musical chairs.

It is a cruel kind of torture to force a nesting woman to see her house in ruins. I try to stave off the anxiety by A) Doing as much as I can by myself and B) Keeping a list.

I have a list of all the things that need to be completed before baba arrives. I look at it every day. It covers what I need for the baby as well as everything that needs to be finished on the house. It's as long as the Great Wall of China.

My mom came over today, helped me spring-clean (I am absolutely enthralled by spring cleaning at the moment) and packed all my stock into the new bookcases in alphabetical order. How I love that woman.

...

I am watching my bump grow from day to day. Am I dreaming?

28 WEEKS

Hospital tour: check.

C-section tentatively booked: check.

Steroids shots: check.

Weekly check-ups: check.

Hospital bag packed: check.

House ready: not even close.

I am using the lounge as an office and we are sleeping in the kitchen. A fine layer of building dust covers absolutely everything in the house, including, among other things: the sleeping cats, the toothbrushes, the bananas in the fruit bowl. We need to use the bathroom tap to fill up the kettle. I get home from my evening walk and Mike and I stand on the exposed beams where the deck is going to be laid, and we talk about buildings and babies.

BERNADETTE HAS ENTERED THE BUILDING

Not knowing when this praevia is going to force an early delivery and the renovation not being close to completion is stressing me out. Stress is bad for baba, I know, and I try to manage it as well as I can, but it is difficult when you are living like a nomad in your own house. Most days I try to ignore the infuriatingly slow pace of the builders, who stand around chatting and laughing in their deep voices. Every day they work at this snail's pace is another day of wages, another day closer to when we will be bringing Mike Jnr home.

Mike had a word with his mom, saying that it's getting too close now, and she has agreed to step in to help finish the house. How I could have kissed her! She has been the project manager on renovations before and is not afraid to give the guys a talking-to. She is quite a thing to behold: petite, made up, and very proper, telling the strong men in overalls that they'd better pull finger, or else. I feel so much better about it. I look at my list again. In this new light, it looks more manageable.

72

THE JIMJAMBOREE

30 WEEKS

Given my contempt for baby showers but really, truly wanting to celebrate this pregnancy and the impending arrival of Mike Jnr, I agreed to having a co-ed PARTY. There was champagne and good food and great company and certainly no belly painting or 'diaper cakes' — ugh! — or games of any kind. We called it the JIMJAMBOREE and Mandie, Pin and Msibi organised it. We had it at Chris's house, as our house is still a building site. He said that not only was it the first baby shower he had ever hosted, but also the first he had ever attended. Mike and I loved it and were awe-struck by the generosity of our friends.

James is already so beloved. I want him to be big and healthy. We've already surpassed the doc's expectations by getting to 30 weeks. I want him to be a big, bonny, vital, chubby baby. Then I'll know we'll be okay. I ate an extra marmite and cheese sandwich, just in case.

32 WEEKS

'So, here's the thing,' says doctor RVR, cracking his knuckles.

Uh-oh, I thought. I've heard that before.

'I'm going to be away for your C-section date.'

'Away?' we both yell. Damn it doc, we want to say. This is no time to go on holiday. This is the most important baby you'll every deliver. Believe us, you'll want to be there! Not on some barge in rural France. Besides, those barges are overrated! And French people are rude. Don't you know anything?

'I'm going in for a back op,' he says.

'A back op?' we say. Now that you say 'back op' it sounds quite serious. We're sure you need the 'back op' but do you really need to have it on the day we're having our Stink Fruit?

'I've been putting it off for 15 years and I can't postpone it any longer.'

'15 years?' we say. 15 years is a long time. You can't possibly postpone it again. That said, if you've already waited 15 years, what difference are a few extra days going to make?

'You'll be in good hands,' he says. Wait a minute, I

think. You were just telling us a few weeks ago that no one else would be able to keep me alive in this surgery. OMG I'm going to die.

'Whose hands?' I ask, expecting a referral to a world-renowned obstetrician of incomparable standing. An obstetrician that has won awards and has a mantelpiece crowded with gynaecologically-themed trophies.

'My wife's,' the doc says.

Ha ha ha! We laugh. What a good joke. 'Funny one, Doc,' we want to say, but our jaws are on the floor and our tongues don't seem to be working.

He's kidding, right? Mike's eyeballs say to me. I hope so, mine say back.

'I'll brief her comprehensively. You'll be fine.'

Who is this 'wife' of yours? we want to ask. Does she even hold a medical degree? And don't say, it's okay, she watches a lot of 'Nurse Jackie' so she kind of knows what she is doing with a scalpel.

Turns out that RVR's wife is an amazingly accomplished obstetrician just down the hallway. Who knew? (Not us). I imagine their home life entails more vagina-speak than most.

34 WEEKS

With maximum two weeks to go until the birth, and the house still in disrepair, I go around sticking up lists like a mad woman. Clear, neat black koki on white sheets, numbered in order of priority. The ceilings are finally going in, the deck should be finished next week. We still don't have water in the kitchen. I have excel spreadsheets — To Do lists for everyone — that gets emailed every day. My OCD is in overdrive, and I'm riding it for all it's worth.

35 WEEKS

We met RVR's 'wife' today, Dr VR, and she seems very proficient. She talked us through the surgery which will hopefully be at 36.3 weeks, on the 5th of April, just in time for the Easter weekend. That's the furtherest we can push it out without tempting the birthing gods with an emergency.

She has been fully briefed by RVR and doesn't think there will be a problem. All the preparations are in place. Forewarned, etc. etc.

We had another look at the baby (hello Cantaloupe!) and he is doing so well and growing so fast. She studied my placenta and also found it hard to believe that I hadn't started bleeding yet. She thanked me for 'being skinny' because it makes her life — or at least, the surgery — a lot easier (so now I know why RVR only wanted me to put on 10kg. Selfish bastard. I could have been eating Nutella ice cream sandwiches for days.) When she said the word 'skinny' I was, like, huh? I don't think supermodels feel skinny at eight months pregnant, and, believe me, I'm no supermodel.

The only thing that worried me was that she said she can only do so much, and the rest is 'in God's hands'. Oh dear, I thought. I'd prefer it if she took a little more responsibility than that. If something goes wrong in the surgery — maybe she'll nick an artery by accident, or maybe I'll just be a bleeder — will she just throw up her arms and say, Oh well, it's God's will? I was hoping, since she was a doctor and all, that she'd be more into science than religion. Dr RVR is the same though. He told me in the beginning that if I had seen what he had seen over his career I would know that miracles do happen.

. . .

Pin came to visit today, bringing more baby stuff, and was horrified by the state of the renovation. I am still working out of the lounge, surrounded by books and boxes. The house is still under a shroud of building dust, despite being cleaned every day. Our bed is in the nursery that I am dying to decorate, but can't until the lights are installed and the dust stops billowing in. The kitchen is still not finished. I am stressed —obviously I am stressed — but am taking it in my stride (I think), although when I saw the concern on her face I thought, Oh Shit. She was worried. She was blinking. I think she may have had tears in her eyes (or maybe it was the paint thinners in the air). It'll be okay, she was saying, clearly not meaning it. So much for nesting, I thought, as I tripped over a box after showing her out.

. . .

I had a full-on argument with the manager of Baby City today over a Sleep Sheep. Yes, A SLEEP SHEEP. Oh the shame, it burns.

...

I'm at the size now that when I sit down in a restaurant the people around me look nervous. You can imagine, then, how people reacted when I was dancing at Jem and Caz's weekend wedding in Muldersdrift. It was wonderful to be away from the house and the To Do lists and so good to be surrounded by friends and family at this (honeydew melon) stage of the pregnancy. I can't believe we have made it this far.

Meeting Mike Jnr is 5 DAYS AWAY.

73

Elastic Vagina

36 weeks

One last scan before the surgery — all is looking good — and little melon is weighing in at 3kg.

I've never understood the whole thing about birth announcements including the weight of the baby. Is it a way of bragging? My baby is bigger/healthier than your baby? Or, 'Look what a massive baby I pushed out!' i.e. Look what an elastic vagina I have!

Surely it is more interesting to hear what colour the baby's hair is, or whose nose he has?

Of course, my puzzlement only applies to full term babies. If you are having a prem then of course the weight is the most important thing. Every gram counts. I didn't think we'd get anywhere close to 3kg.

74

BIRTH STORY

I am sitting here on my hospital bed with the most beautiful baby ever born. He is fed and swaddled and sleeping with the most peaceful expression on his (adorable) old man/monkey face. The room smells of birth and babies: colostrum and vernix. The surgery went without a hitch, apart from one 'bleeder!' that was quickly fixed. I have decided that I have a crush on doctor VR. She was amazing. It went so well that I am back in the maternity ward and didn't have to be moved to ICU, which I am so grateful for because it means I can lie with this precious little boy on my chest for hours and hours and hours. I never want to let him go. I may keep him here forever, or at least until he is a teenager.

The birth was everything I had imagined and more. Having a real live baby is mind-blowingly wonderful. I have never felt so deeply satisfied in my life. I feel like I am radiating joy. I feel like I have a golden glow about me: Madonna and child.

I struggled a bit with the pain earlier — I wasn't given the pethidine shot I was supposed to get in recovery so it rushed at me before I knew what was happening and I lay paralysed and sweating before the paed saw my condition and ordered drugs. That was the only difficult part of the day. Now here I sit, stitched up, drugged up, and completely under the spell of this miraculous child. I can't imagine ever being sad again.

It is a tradition on the FC forum to post your birth story once you have had your little one. I also wanted to get the details down so that I could remember them later when the fuzziness wears off, and, of course, to send to the Mike Jnr Fan club. (Oh! Before I forget: he was born weighing 2.6kg). Here it is:

After a lovely Last Supper up the road and a near sleepless night, our alarms went off at 4am on the 5th of April. It was finally the day to meet our little boy! We rushed to Sandton Mediclinic (you would swear by Mike's driving that I was in an advanced stage of labour and in danger of giving birth right there in the passenger seat — but I wasn't complaining) and were shown to a private ward (we had been inexplicably upgraded) – further proof that it was to be the luckiest day of my life – and sat around not sure what to do and smiling a lot.

There was paperwork to be filled out and although I didn't feel too nervous I must have been as I made so many mistakes that I had to fill out the same form twice. I told the nurse I was 29 (I'm 32) and that my blood group was O+ (it's O-).

There was a tiny baby-sized hospital gown next to

mine: it was so small and cute it almost melted my face. Mike looked dashing in his scrubs and held my (clammy) hand while the docs set to work. There were grins all round, mine the widest.

The anaesthetist was excellent: he explained everything in detail beforehand and the spinal block wasn't as nearly as painful as I expected it to be. Then the catheter was in and the surgeon was checking the block had worked, and before I could get too nervous they had already started cutting. It was the strangest sensation: I could feel them cutting and rummaging and applying pressure, but there was no pain. They didn't put a screen up, which sounds gory but was wonderful because I got to see my son the moment he was lifted out of me.

One minute I was pregnant, the next there was a beautiful baby boy.

Seeing him for the first time was the most intense, full-on emotional high I have ever experienced. He let out a lusty yell and we laughed (and cried). It felt unreal and super-real at the same time. The paed checked him, called him 'beautiful' a couple of times, and placed him high up on my chest. Mike had his head next to mine and the three of us huddled and looked at each other and laughed and cried some more.

I didn't want to think about my fertility issues today, but all the previous hope and heartbreak was there in the room with me and when I saw that sweet, pink, fragrant little body it felt like my heart was bursting. Every disappointment, every loss, every shard of pain turned into an overwhelming feeling of love and joy.

It was a completely mind-blowing, soul-bending experience, and more than anything I could have imagined.

75

THE HAPPINESS FACTORY

We brought James home today. (Still dreaming?) The cats greeted him, as expected, with remarkable indifference. The house is dust-free and filled with flowers and easter eggs. I am walking on clouds. We sit outside on the new deck and drink tea and eat chocolate. Friends and family come to fawn and feed us. They always exclaim at how tiny James is. Chris held him today — we have a lovely photo — and he does look minuscule in his arms. We'll frame the pic and give it to him as a gift when we are semi-functioning adults again.

I spend almost all day breastfeeding. James yells for milk every 2 hours or so. I think that he knows he is prem and is trying to catch up. Like a typical newborn, he doesn't do much more than eat and sleep. Mike calls my (huge) boobs 'The Happiness Factory'.

The sleep deprivation is tough going but Mike and I have had plenty of training in advertising all-nighters.

We are tag-teaming like never before. Nappies, burp cloths, tiny little onesies, tea, cookies. When we are feeling less exhausted we watch series together (Game of Thrones; Downton Abbey), eat pizza and share a beer (Yes! Beer! He started drinking again the night James was born, praise the gods).

When we are worn out we stumble across each others' paths, grunting in greeting, like (grumpy) ships in the night. We can go a whole day without looking each other in the eyes. He cradles James and sings to him and I've never loved him more.

The C-section wound is sore, but having James makes it less so. The most painful part is sitting up in bed at night, to feed him, but as soon as I have him in my arms and he is guzzling away (there really is no other word for the way he eats) I get to think: this is real. He is real. He is mine (although I know that he is not *mine*-mine, but he is the most mine he'll ever be).

Dear James

These are some of the things I love about you:

1. The way you open your mouth wide when it's time to eat, and shake your head from side to side. Then you chomp down like as if you're taking a big bite out of a cheeseburger.

2. Your latch, always surprising in its vacuum power. You're like an especially endearing Electrolux.

3. The way you kick in the bath.

4. Your eternal eyes.

5. The way you're so frowny and serious even though you're still so tiny.

6. The way you burp (like a champion).

7. No matter how upset you are beforehand, you always settle down when I put you on my chest.

8. How cute you look swaddled. We call you our beautiful Breakfast Burrito.

9. How, when you are feeding, you are so noisy: lip smacking, gulping, wheezing, grunting. And how sometimes you put your arms up, as if in surrender.

10. The way you splay your toes.

11. How when you are really hungry you gum anything near your mouth: burp cloth, blanket, and your special favourite: the head support in your pram.

12. How your skin changes colour, like a gecko.

13. Your downy blond barely-there hair, even though you seemed to get my hair and your Dad's hairline, which is the exact opposite of what we ordered.

14. I love the way you, weekly and without fail, pee on the baby clinic nurse. Not because I don't like the nurse, just because I find it adorable, and a little bit eccentric.

...

People have been asking if having a newborn is difficult. Yes and no, I say. The good parts are better than the bad parts are bad. Yes, you're in absolute survivor mode, but you are buoyed by this delightful creature that needs you 24/7. Sometimes you feel as though the delightful creature is draining the very life out of you. A delightful baby vampire. You give everything you have but the baby needs more than that, so you give that, too. You're running on love and oxytocin and chocolate and the realisation that you have at last realised your dream. You think that you want time to yourself, to wash your hair and get things done, but you miss him as soon as you put him down to sleep. You miss him so much that instead of doing the laundry and catching up on work you find yourself looking at pictures of him on your phone. Finally you see the reason for Instagram to exist.

Is having a newborn difficult? Not for me. At least: it's not as difficult as infertility. Not even close.

76

CHOCOLATE DRAWER

Today I boxed up all the painkillers that were in my bedside table drawer. Before infertility it had been my sex drawer, then it became my TTC drawer (thermometers, temperature charts, pre-seed) and then my pain drawer (pills and little black book of pain). Now, I am very happy to announce, it has become my chocolate drawer. My life is complete. Any breastfeeding woman will tell you that tea and chocolate in copious amounts are the absolute staples in any BF diet. As James was born during Easter we have kilograms of chocolate to get through. Mike bought James his first Easter egg: it was almost the same size as him. I helped eat it.

77

A Happy Beginning

This journal has been essential to my beating infertility. It has allowed me to process every fear, and every hope. It's allowed me to laugh a bit along the way, too, to try to look at the comical side when long days and nights were anything but. (Mike always says I laugh at my own jokes. I say, of course I do! I wouldn't tell jokes that I didn't think were funny.)

When I turn back and read how I was feeling three years ago, when this tortuous (and sometimes torturous) journey started, I see how far I have come. If only I could have used the flux capacitor to go back in time and tell my younger self that I WOULD eventually fall pregnant and have a baby — an absolutely beautiful, healthy, delicious baby — it would have made the trip so much easier. It was the not knowing that was the worst.

I wish I could have told myself: Don't worry about the money. There is always More Money. Don't worry about the business or the energy or the way infertility drains your very lifeblood. Keep working, but don't worry. There is always more lifeblood (until there's not, and then you'll be dead and you won't have to worry about anything anyway).

Don't worry about that old grey face that stares back at you in the mirror. It will get better. There is not necessarily always a dream (or baby) realised unless you do everything in your power to make it happen. Don't worry about being 'obsessed' or that you find it all-consuming. Accept that it IS all-consuming. Sometimes you need to be consumed. Sometimes you do have to push. Sometimes you have to push harder. It's worth it. It's worth it. It couldn't be more worth it.

It's time to sign off now and put this journal away. It's finished. It's time to start a new one, about James and Mike and our new upside-down life together. There are new memories (and new notes) to be made. Bright and sweet. As they say in dodgy Thai spas the world over: Now it's time for the Happy Ending. And as with all happy endings, it's not really an ending at all, at its heart, but a happy beginning.

ACKNOWLEDGMENTS

Thanks go to my editor, Bronwen Muller,
for whipping this manuscript into shape.

Thanks also go to my Dad, Keith Thiele,
and his better half, Gillian,
for proofreading every story I write, even when
I give them impossible deadlines (and the rugby's on).

Thank you to my wonderful beta readers: Priscilla Fick;
Kim Smith; Fiona Coward; Angelique Pacheco; Chelsea
Humphrey and Janice Leibowitz.

Most of all, thanks go to my husband, Mike,
who not only supported me in our struggle with infertility,
but helped me prepare this book for print,
along with another eleventy thousand things.
Thank you, I love you.
#tagteamoflove

ALSO BY JT LAWRENCE

The Memory of Water (2011)

Why You Were Taken (2015)

Sticky Fingers (2016)

Grey Magic (2016)

How We Found You (2017)

ABOUT THE AUTHOR

JT Lawrence is an author, playwright
& bookdealer. She lives in Parkhurst, Johannesburg,
in a house with a red front door.

STAY IN TOUCH

If you'd like to be notified of giveaways
& new releases, sign up for JT Lawrence's mailing list
via Facebook or on her author platform at
https://pulpbooks.wordpress.com/

Printed in Great Britain
by Amazon